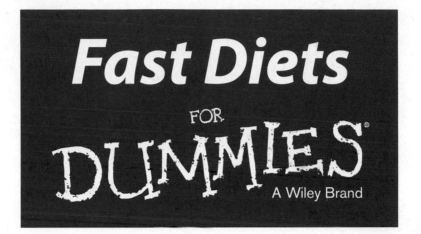

Fast Diets
FOR
DUMMIES®
A Wiley Brand

by Kellyann Petrucci, MD, and Patrick Flynn
Authors of *Paleo Workouts For Dummies*

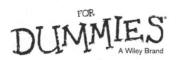

FOR
DUMMIES®
A Wiley Brand

Fast Diets For Dummies®

Published by: **John Wiley & Sons, Inc.,** 111 River Street, Hoboken, NJ 07030-5774, www.wiley.com

Copyright © 2014 by John Wiley & Sons, Inc., Hoboken, New Jersey

Published simultaneously in Canada

Library of Congress Control Number: 2013949525

ISBN: 978-1-118-77508-0

ISBN 978-1-118-77295-3 (ebk); ISBN 978-1-118-77509-7 (ebk); ISBN 978-1-118-77510-3 (ebk)

Manufactured in the United States of America

10 9 8 7 6 5 4 3 2 1

Contents at a Glance

Table of Contents

Introduction

$\textbf{\textit{W}}$elcome to the world of fasting. In fact, fasting is the world's oldest cure-all. Hippocrates, the father of medicine, once said "instead of medicine, fast for a day." What's more, all animals, except the modern-day human, fast instinctively when sick or injured. The healing power of fasting has been known for all time, of that there is no doubt, but it hasn't been until recently that people in the fields of fitness, health, nutrition, and healing have had the science to back it up.

We wrote this book to bring fasting back to the forefront — as a healing mechanism, as a fat loss booster, as a muscle builder, and more.

Now it doesn't matter whether or not you want to drop a few pounds, heal a disease, fight aging, or enhance vitality, fasting can give it all to you, whether you want it or not. The benefits are enormous and they're inescapable.

About This Book

Fast Diets For Dummies gives you all you ever wanted to know about fasting, which simply means not eating for a while. That doesn't sound too difficult, right? Surely anyone could figure out on his or her own that the way to do so is not to put food in your mouth.

For some reason though, it's not easy. Many people are overweight, unhealthy, and sick. Fasting is a delicate art. Subtle nuances can make or break a fast, and little tweaks can diminish or enhance the positive effects of fasting.

In addition, you can go about fasting in numerous ways. Some of them are more difficult than others, no doubt, but each serves a distinctly unique purpose. For example, some methods of fasting are better suited for putting on muscle, other methods for burning fat.

Fast Diets For Dummies can help you find the best fasting protocol for you, as well as help ease you gently into the process. Fasting can be tough — we're not going to hide that — but know that with disciplined effort, the reward is great.

This book is different from any other available fasting book, because we aren't emotionally (or financially) tied to any one practice or organization. What you have here is an unbiased and honest overview of some of the more popular fasting protocols around today. Our job is to help you sift through the garbage, find the gold, take it, and run.

In this book, we provide two chapters, chock-full of recipes. One chapter provides 500-calorie meals and the other has 600-calorie meals for your one meal that you eat, depending on the fast you choose to follow. (Part II discusses the different fasting options.) Here are some general conventions that we use in the recipes:

- ✔ Milk is whole.
- ✔ Eggs are large.
- ✔ Pepper is freshly ground black pepper unless otherwise specified.
- ✔ Butter is unsalted.
- ✔ Flour is all-purpose unless otherwise specified.
- ✔ Sugar is granulated unless otherwise noted.
- ✔ All herbs are fresh unless dried herbs are specified.
- ✔ All temperatures are Fahrenheit.

If you need to convert the recipes into metric measurements, check out www.dummies.com/how-to/content/dealing-with-metric-measurements.html for help.

Foolish Assumptions

When writing this book, we made the following assumptions about you:

- ✔ You want to improve your general condition or specifically one condition. Perhaps you want to be healthier, leaner, or more productive. Perhaps you want to be all three.
- ✔ You want to lose weight.
- ✔ You have tried diets in the past and been dissatisfied with the results or frustrated with the process.

Fast Diets For Dummies shows you how to lose weight, improve your overall health and well-being, and have more energy, all quickly, safely, and without all the pains of conventional dieting. We want to make this life-changing process as enjoyable as possible.

Icons Used in This Book

Throughout this book, and in true *For Dummies* fashion, you'll run into a number of icons — all of them designed to help you better understand and get the most out of intermittent fasting. Here are the icons you can expect to run into throughout this book:

This icon provides helpful information that you can implement in your fasting.

This icon points out important tidbits that you should store in your mind because you'll probably end up revisiting them in your fasting endeavors.

We don't post warnings often, but when we do, pay attention, because they're enormously important. Don't skip over them unless you want to fall into a potentially harmful mistake.

This text discusses the nitty-gritty and often scientific details about certain concepts. This information isn't essential to your fast, but certainly recommended!

This icon directs you to additional free information you can find online to help you with your fast.

Beyond the Book

In addition to all the information in *Fast Diets For Dummies,* you can find additional information online to help you with your fast. We provide a free Cheat Sheet online at www.dummies.com/cheatsheet/fastdiets. The Cheat Sheet adds a few extra tidbits that you will find interesting. You can also find additional information online at www.dummies.com/extras/fastdiets.

If after reading the Cheat Sheet and online information, you want more, you can then check out our own websites:

✔ www.chroniclesofstrength.com: Pat's website is based around the philosophy of fitness minimalism and offers a plethora of unconventional fasting protocols and super-efficient strength and conditioning routines.

✔ www.drkellyann.com: This website is your one-stop Paleo Shop, offering you everything you need to know about what to eat when you're not fasting (which is equally important to the practice of fasting itself) and what not to eat.

Where to Go from Here

All you need to start is an open mind. Much of the information you're about to encounter in this book is in stark opposition to conventional wisdom. And because the majority of people aren't yet on board with fasting, it remains a bit controversial.

But just remember what Mark Twain said, "Whenever you find yourself on the side of the majority, it's time to pause and reflect."

Consider this book a fasting buffet (ironic, we know). Take from it what you will; you don't need to read it cover to cover unless you want a good and thorough understanding on the subject matter. Nor do we require you to memorize anything. After you find what you need, you can let this book sit ready on your shelf for you to pick up anytime you need a quick refresher.

You can start from Chapter 1 and read to the end, or you can flip to the Table of Contents or the index to find a topic that interests you. You can read just the chapters or sections that interest you. No matter what you read, we wish you luck in your fasting lifestyle change.

Part I
Getting Started with Fast Diets

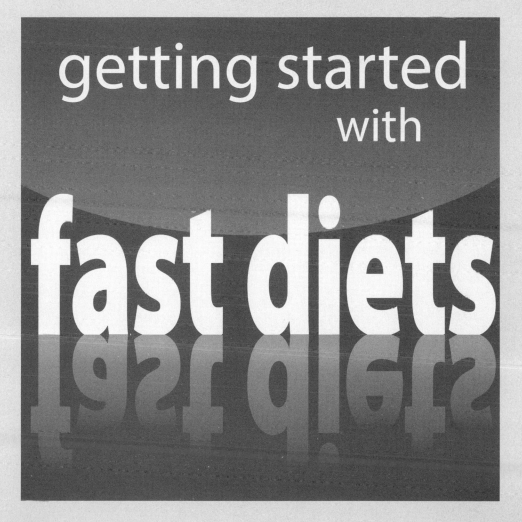

 Visit www.dummies.com/extras/fastdiets for more helpful great Dummies content online.

In this part...

- Examine the science behind fasting and why your body won't go into starvation mode (or in other words, hold on to body fat and feel lethargic) while you fast.

- Understand the many benefits of fasting and how fasting can improve, not just your physical health, such as muscle gain, immunity, and fat loss, but also your neurological health, including brain function and productivity.

- Find out how exercising while in a fasted state is so powerful for burning fat and building muscle.

- See how having the proper mindset and setting realistic expectations can make your experiences with fasting more successful.

- Discover techniques that can help you overcome any fasting pitfalls so that you can utilize fasting to its fullest potential.

Chapter 1

Fasting — Nature's Ultimate Fat-Burning Secret Weapon

. . . .

In This Chapter

▶ Discovering what fasting is

▶ Understanding what fasting can do for you

▶ Recognizing who should and shouldn't fast

▶ Determining whether or not fasting is right for you

. . . .

*A*lmost any diet works, for a period of time. Because at root, all diets operate on the same premises — calorie restriction. Though many try to deny this plain and simple fact, it's quite undeniable. If you take in fewer calories than you get rid of, you will lose weight. It's inevitable.

You don't need to eat healthy to lose weight, believe it or not. You need only to eat less. But we don't recommend that you cut your intake of sandwich cookies in half, from ten to five, because being healthy is more than just losing weight. In other words you can be thin and unhealthy.

A good diet is an economical one. It contains no unnecessary foods and no unnecessary meals, which means you're judicious about your food quality and also your food quantity. As a result, you should omit needless foods, which means anything you ingest that that will either make you more or less healthy. If a food doesn't directly benefit you, then you should omit it. Many good books discuss the importance of food quality. (In this book, we briefly discuss food quality, but our mission is to focus on quantity.)

This chapter (and this book) focuses on the quantity — how to not eat — in other words, how to fast for health, fat loss, and longevity. Not eating, in fact, is darn near one of the healthiest things you can do for yourself that you've probably never thought to do. And you've probably never thought to do it, because all conventional wisdom has led you to believe that skipping meals or not eating for a while is bad for you.

In this chapter we introduce you to fasting to help you understand what fasting is, why it's such a beneficial health practice, and why it's so darn effective for weight loss. We then help you decide whether or not fasting is right for you.

Getting a Better Idea of What Fasting Really Is

The concept of fasting is quite simple. *Fasting* means you don't eat for a while. Although it may sound a bit contrarian, it is, without a doubt, a very safe and very sound health practice. In fact, it's good for your mind, body, and soul.

You may have heard that not eating is a bad idea, because it will slow your metabolism and cause you to gain weight. Well, you've heard wrong. Fasting is not only good for you, but also perhaps the healthiest thing you can ever do for yourself.

Fasting works because it's a hardship. It's short-term deprivation, to be exact. And, to that end, any diet that touts itself as superior because it isn't deprivation-based is not superior at all, but far inferior, to be sure. Any diet that says you can "eat whatever you want so long as you . . . " or "eat as much as you want so long as you . . . " is immediately a pile of fatuous nonsense and is to be straightaway ignored.

These sections examine the positive benefits of fasting, explain how fasting works, and discuss how you can fast. The other chapters in Part I provide more detail about these discussions to help if you want to change your lifestyle for the better and incorporate fasting into your diet.

Identifying the positive effects of fasting

Fasting can help you feel and look better. In addition, here are a few of the positive effects fasting can have on your body. Fasting

✔ **Burns fat:** When fasting, the body naturally taps into stored body fat for energy, a process that is severely inhibited when eating frequently throughout the day. Studies have shown that fasting dramatically increases *lipolysis,* which is the fancy term for fat burning.

✔ **Boosts energy:** Fasting is slightly stimulatory, because it increases your natural adrenal response. In plain English, it means that while you're fasting, you can expect your productivity to increase and concentration to improve.

✔ **Fights disease:** Fasting naturally boosts immunity and allows your body to naturally detoxify itself. While fasting, your body purges unhealthy, damaged, and polluted cells — as well as spurs the growth of new healthy cells.

✔ **Delays aging:** Eating has an aging effect on the body, which happens primarily through *insulin,* which is your body's primary nutrient transport and blood-sugar regulating hormone. When you eat, your pancreas secretes insulin. And the problem with eating too much or too frequently is that insulin speeds up biological aging process. Fasting delays aging by suppressing insulin levels.

✔ **Enhances exercise:** Fasting and exercise potentiate each other, meaning they increase each other's positive effects. Exercising in a fasted state can help you to burn more fat, increase vitality, and build muscle more efficiently.

The benefits of fasting are huge, whereas there really isn't a reason why you shouldn't fast on a regular basis. In fact, fasting is also the world's most ancient healing mechanism. All animals, except human beings, fast instinctively when sick or wounded. Chapter 2 discusses these benefits in more detail.

Examining how it works

The human body can be either in a fasted state or a fed state; it can't be in between. Therefore, if the fed state is yang, then the fasting state is yin. Fasting provides balance — by adding in more yin to counterweigh all that yang. Fasting basically works in three ways:

✔ **It optimizes your hormonal makeup.** When in a fasted state, hormones that are particularly beneficial are permitted free reign, including *glucagon,* which is the yin to insulin's yang. Glucagon, like insulin, is secreted by the pancreas in order to regulate blood sugar. But rather than shutting nutrients into cells, glucagon pulls nutrients out of cells, including fatty acids, which has earned glucagon the reputation of being something of a fat-burning hormone. However, glucagon can only prevail in a fasted state.

✔ **It surges natural growth hormone.** Insulin, the hormone secreted during the fed state, heavily suppresses natural growth hormone. Meaning, the more frequently you eat, the less natural growth hormone your body produces. Natural growth hormone is the closest thing humans have to a fountain of youth. It burns fat, builds muscle, and works to keep the body biologically young and resilient.

✔ **It permits the body to cleanse itself.** When in a fasted state, the body disperses its natural house cleaners, which consist primarily of *microphages* (think of these as cells that attack and destroy harmful invaders) and white blood cells that pull toxins out of cells, engulf them, and dispose of them. When constantly fed, this natural detoxification process is hampered. Frequently feeding functions as a one-way escape valve, permitting toxins into the body, but not letting them back out. Not until you enter a fasted state can you flip that valve and allow toxins to pour out of the body.

Chapter 2 delves deeper into the science of fasting.

Understanding the best way to go about it

You may be surprised to hear that you can go about fasting in several different ways. Some of them include longer fasting periods (up to 24 hours at a time), whereas others include short fasting periods (12 to 16 hours). Some methods include strict fasts (nothing but water) and others include controlled fasts (limited caloric intake).

In this book, we discuss four common fasting options. These options are as follows:

✔ **Intermittent fasting:** Intermittent fasting is when you fast for 24 to 36 hours (typically once or twice a week). This method is a simple way to introduce fasting into your life because you only need to take a break from eating for a day. This works exceptionally well to reduce overall calorie intake without having to worry about making many other changes on your nonfasting days. Check out Chapter 4 for more details.

✔ **5:2 Diet:** The 5:2 Diet, also known as the Fast Diet, is the gentlest introduction to fasting, because it simply requires that for two days out of the week you only eat two meals (500-calorie meals if you're a woman and 600-calorie meals if you're a man). This method is perhaps the best way for most people to get acclimated with fasting, before perusing some of the more intensive efforts. Chapter 5 gives you the lowdown on this method.

✔ **Micro-fasting:** Micro-fasting is a daily fasting regimen. Think of it as the no breakfast diet. This idea flies in the face of conventional wisdom, but for good reasons (all of which we explain in Chapter 6). Micro-fasting has you fasting for 16 hours each day, compressing the time you eat into an eight-hour window. Micro-fasting is both easy to implement and enormously beneficial. Head to Chapter 6 for how to incorporate micro-fasting into your diet.

✔ **The Warrior Diet:** The Warrior Diet, made popular by the book of the same title, is similar to micro-fasting in the sense that it condenses the time you're allowed to eat into a small window (about four hours), but different in a few other regards. The fasting period is less strict, and more of a controlled fast, where you're encouraged to consume certain live/raw foods throughout the earlier parts of the day followed by a fairly intense overeating phase later in the day. The Warrior Diet is unconventional, effective, and satisfying. Chapter 7 explains the ins and outs of the Warrior Diet.

Understanding the best way to fast is simply a matter of preference. All fasts work, and each has its unique benefits. Our job, in this book, is to explain and to review these four popular and effective fasting protocols and then to help you select the one that best fits your lifestyle. The best fasting method for you is the one that you will stick to. The method you choose is little concern of ours. We just want you to choose one and then stick to it.

Tapping into the roots of fasting: No carrots involved

Fasting goes back thousands and thousands of years to ancient Greece. The Greeks were fond of fasting for its ability to clarify the mind and purify the body. Hippocrates, the father of western medicine, advocated fasting as a preventive measure as well as a prescription to remedy all serious ailments.

The famous Greek historian Plutarch once wrote, "Instead of medicine, rather, fast a day."

Many other wise men of days long past recognized fasting's amazing restorative abilities.

Plato and Aristotle also encouraged fasting to enhance physical well-being and boost mental prowess.

Great men also practiced fasting from other cultures. Buddha liked fasting. And so did Jesus.

If only humankind knew now what it did back then, which is the simple notion that the body thrives under hardship. The difficulties in life don't kill, but the pleasures — drunkenness, idleness, and gluttony to name a few — do.

Figuring Out Why People Should Fast

Fasting is something you should do from time to time, even if you're not trying to lose weight. The general health benefits of fasting are simply too enormous to ignore.

People who fast regularly experience the following:

- A lower risk of diseases, such as diabetes, heart disease, cancer, Alzheimer's disease, and Parkinson's disease
- Improved cognitive function
- A leaner physique

Quite plainly, fasting is, before anything else, a practice for health and longevity. And to know whether or not you should fast is merely a matter of answering the question "Do I want to live longer and healthier?" If the answer is yes, then you should fast.

Many people may want to consider fasting with the intention of losing some weight, so these sections examine why fasting is a no-brainer if you're looking to get leaner.

Losing weight equals calorie restriction

In order to lose weight, you have to take in fewer calories than you use. All diets — low-fat diets, low-carb diets, whatever diet, at the end of the day — all aim to achieve the same objective — a calorie deficit — which explains why just about any diet will work for a period of time. How fasting and all the other diets differ is that fasting is perhaps the safest, healthiest, and quickest way to assume a calorie deficit.

Not all diets are healthy, as you probably know, and being healthy is a lot more than just losing weight. A good, healthy diet is a balanced diet comprised of high-quality food sources, including meat, seafood, nuts, vegetables, and fruit. A healthy diet avoids heavily processed or man-made food sources, because even though they may cause you to lose weight, they pollute your system with harmful additives and chemicals.

Chapter 8 identifies the healthful types of foods you can eat, no matter whether you're on a fast or during your off-fast times.

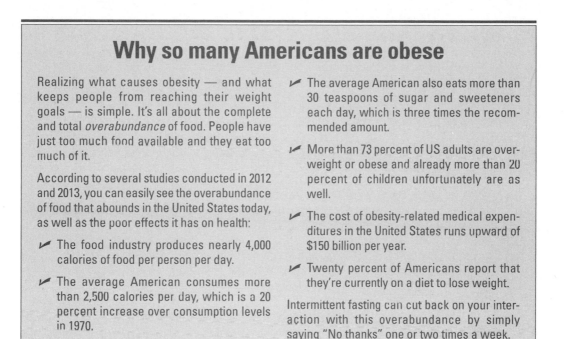

Why so many Americans are obese

Realizing what causes obesity — and what keeps people from reaching their weight goals — is simple. It's all about the complete and total *overabundance* of food. People have just too much food available and they eat too much of it.

According to several studies conducted in 2012 and 2013, you can easily see the overabundance of food that abounds in the United States today, as well as the poor effects it has on health:

✔ The food industry produces nearly 4,000 calories of food per person per day.

✔ The average American consumes more than 2,500 calories per day, which is a 20 percent increase over consumption levels in 1970.

✔ The average American also eats more than 30 teaspoons of sugar and sweeteners each day, which is three times the recommended amount.

✔ More than 73 percent of US adults are overweight or obese and already more than 20 percent of children unfortunately are as well.

✔ The cost of obesity-related medical expenditures in the United States runs upward of $150 billion per year.

✔ Twenty percent of Americans report that they're currently on a diet to lose weight.

Intermittent fasting can cut back on your interaction with this overabundance by simply saying "No thanks" one or two times a week.

Burning calories becomes easier

Fasting is at root all about creating a calorie deficit. And fasting makes it easy. Fasting takes large chunks out of your weekly calorie intake. And it does so fairly painlessly too. For example, say right now you consume about 2,000 calories to maintain your current weight, which is 14,000 calories a week. If you implement one full 24-hour fast once a week, your weekly caloric intake is reduced to 12,000 calories.

Will reducing your weekly caloric intake by 2,000 calories cause you to lose weight? Of course! The best part is that you didn't need to worry about counting calories or changing anything else. All you had to do was take a break from eating for a day. If you eat the Paleo Diet (see Chapter 8 for more details) on your nonfasting days, which we highly recommend, you will not only be able to reduce caloric intake further, if you choose, but you'll also take solace knowing that you're fueling your body with the foods you were designed to eat, the foods that promote health at a cellular level.

What makes fasting so powerful is that it does what other diets aim to do (reduce calories) quicker and with far less torment. Yes, skipping meals is still the best way to go about losing weight — always has been, always will be. There is no easier way to assume a calorie deficit than fasting.

Just remember that fasting won't make up for an otherwise terrible diet. You should use fasting in combination with a sound, healthful diet, such as the Paleo Diet, for maximum effects. For more on the Paleo Diet, please check out our other book, *Living Paleo For Dummies* (John Wiley & Sons, Inc.).

Determining who should and shouldn't fast

Fasting has been known to help alleviate and reverse many chronic health conditions, such as inflammation, Type-2 diabetes, and hypertension. However, fasting may not be right for everybody right away.

Before you start any fasting protocol, consult your doctor. If you have any health issues that you think may be aggravated by fasting, be sure to discuss them with your doctor as well. And feel free to bring this book to your next visit and discuss the various fasting options with your doctor, so that he or she can also help you to decide if fasting is right for you, and if so, which fasting course is the best fit for you.

The following lists different categories of people and whether fasting may or may not be right for them:

- **Healthy adults:** All healthy adults should engage in some sort of fast from time to time. There is no reason not to, and fasting may be the very thing that keeps them healthy.

- **Children:** Most children, up to the age of 18, don't need to fast. Although most children shouldn't eat as frequently as they do, they need not engage in prolonged bouts of fasting. Children are growing and need sound nutrition to do so.

  The exception to this rule is overweight children. The first step in reversing childhood obesity shouldn't be fasting, but instead restructuring their diet. Get the child eating healthily first, removing all sugar and junk food. After a child is eating healthily, you'll likely find it unnecessary to also have him or her fast. But, as always, if you're under the age of 18 or have a child who you believe might benefit from fasting, consult with your doctor first.

- **People with Type-2 Diabetes:** Fasting has been used for ages as a means to help reverse Type-2 diabetes, and the research on its effectiveness to do so is astonishing. However, if you have Type-2 diabetes, you must absolutely consult with your doctor before engaging in any sort of fasting protocol.

- **Immunosuppressed individuals:** Any individual who is immunosuppressed, such as someone with HIV/AIDS, cancer, lupus, or anything similar, must consult with his or her doctor before engaging in any sort of fasting protocol.

✔ **Pregnant women:** Studies on the effects of fasting on pregnant women during Ramadan have indicated no negative effects on mother or child. But just like any other special circumstance, if you're pregnant and want to fast, you must first garner your doctor's approval.

✔ **High-level athletes:** High-level athletes too can benefit from fasting. Fasting helps to enhance recovery and improve nutrient-uptake efficiency, which makes the muscle-building and strength-gaining processes easier. But a high-level athlete must judiciously apply fasting. Don't fast on game days or before any other circumstance where you require a substantial amount of gas in the tank.

✔ **People with eating disorders:** People with eating disorders should consult with a psychotherapist. Although fasting is very healthful, it won't cure the underlying emotional disorder as related to food.

✔ **Vegans or vegetarians:** Fasting can be implemented with nearly any form of diet or lifestyle. It's particularly suitable for vegans and vegetarians as well.

Asking Yourself Whether It's Right for You

Fasting is right for anyone seeking a longer, healthier, and more vibrant life. However, you may have a few other questions that you want answered to help you determine whether fasting is right for you. Here are some common questions and answers to help you make that important decision:

✔ **How well do you manage hunger?** When you fast, you'll get hungry. Unfortunately it's unavoidable. What will make you successful is your ability to manage hunger, embrace it even. If you know that you're a person who simply can't tolerate any hunger of any kind (which is an issue for you to figure out why), fasting can help you get a handle on it. Fasting teaches you how to not let hunger control you. Chapter 14 provides ten quick ways to help you battle hunger when you're fasting.

✔ **Are you willing to commit to at least three months?** Nothing works immediately. And frankly, if you're not willing to commit to a fasting protocol for three solid months, without deviation, then you're just not giving it a fair shot. Note that after three months, you don't just stop. Fasting is a lifestyle — a permanent change. Three months is simply the test-drive period to fairly assess whether or not fasting is right for you. We hope you incorporate it into your diet for the rest of your life.

- ✔ **Can you focus and get into the right mindset?** Fasting requires a certain degree of mental toughness and fortitude. Fasting, like exercise, is a stressor. And mild stressors, such as fasting and exercise, are required to maintain optimum health, so don't enter fasting expecting it to be a pleasure cruise. Nothing worthwhile is ever a pleasure cruise, except for, of course, an actual pleasure cruise, but even most of those are overrated. For you to be successful, you must first expect to be challenged. If being challenged doesn't sound like something you want, then fasting probably isn't right for you.

- ✔ **How is your diet otherwise?** Fasting won't save you from an otherwise unhealthy diet. Before you begin a fasting protocol, make sure you get your diet in order. To get the most from fasting, you need to eat healthily when not fasting. We recommend the Paleo Diet, which is a diet based on how your ancestors used to eat, comprised mostly of meats, seafood, nuts, vegetables, and fruit, while omitting sugar, flour, and grains. Check out Chapter 8 for more details about the Paleo Diet.

- ✔ **What do you think of exercise?** To get the most out of fasting, you need to incorporate some form of exercise into your life. Indeed you can fast without exercising, but you'll be missing out on the full spectrum of physical and mental benefits if you do. Fasting and exercise actually work to boost the benefits of each other. We provide you with sample exercise routines in this book (check out Chapter 12) to help get you started combining fasting and exercise. For a more complete guide on how to properly exercise for maximum impact, please check out our book *Paleo Workouts For Dummies* (John Wiley & Sons, Inc.).

- ✔ **How is your lifestyle otherwise?** Fasting can do some amazing things. It can heal conditions, boost immunity, burn fat, and increase productivity. But fasting is best served in conjunction with other healthy habits. Before beginning a fasting protocol, we recommend that you also introduce other healthy habits into lifestyle as well, such as physical exercise, because fasting works to boost all the positive effects of exercise. Refer to the chapters in Part 4 for more on exercise and other healthy lifestyle habits that are important.

- ✔ **Do you have a support system?** When starting something such a as new diet or exercise program, people tend to adhere for longer and more strictly when they begin with a friend, family member, or colleague. Before embarking on your fasting journey, seek out someone who might wish to join you, so that you can hold each other accountable. This is an effective way to ensure progress. To get the most out of your support system, force each other to keep a food journal, detailing your fasting periods and everything else you eat throughout the week. Chapter 3 discusses how to rely on your support system.

What gets measured gets managed. Keeping a food journal forces you to think twice before you put something into your mouth. It often helps deter you from making poor food choices, even if you don't have a support system to share the food journal. If keeping a full food log of everything you eat throughout the week sounds like too much, then snap a picture of it on your phone before you eat it. Doing so can make you think twice before putting junk food into your mouth.

If you decide to fast, check out www.dummies.com/extras/fastdiets for a bonus Part of Tens list for some tricks to help you get the most from your fast.

How I started fasting: Pat Flynn

I'm a minimalist. In almost all circumstances, I believe that less equals more, which has been my philosophy on exercise for a number of years now and what makes me a little bit different. And because I am a man who is incessantly seeking efficiency, I always strive to do the least amount I need to do to get the job done, and not a smidgen more.

In other words, I believe any exercise program will improve in direct ratio to the number of things kept out of it that needn't be there. I now say the exact same thing about nutrition. Basically any nutrition program will improve in direct ratio to the number of things kept out of it that needn't be there, which means, of course, to omit any needless meals, foods, and supplements.

I was introduced to fasting five years ago, when a colleague of mine handed me a book about the Warrior Diet. He challenged me to stick to it for three months, despite my skepticism. I did and my results were spectacular. My daily energy levels soared while my body fat levels plummeted. I felt enervated, more alive than ever before, as if a deep fog had been lifted that I never even knew existed until it was gone.

I spent the next four years researching and experimenting the miracle of fasting. And I couldn't believe how wrong everything I ever thought I knew about nutrition up to that point had been. The research on fasting is clear and astounding. The benefits are enormous. Yet people are lead to believe, through various media manipulators (namely large food corporations) that not eating is somewhat deleterious. This, of course, is ridiculous. It's just not true.

Fasting changed my life, and I am deeply appreciative that I got such an early start on it. I now keep 7 to 8 percent body fat year-round, and very rarely do I ever eat before noon. I'm healthier than ever before (and yes, I have the blood work to prove it), more productive, and an all-around happier person. All because of fasting.

My chief aim now is to share with you the power of fasting — to help you implement fasting into your life, so that you can start to make the progress that you deserve to make. I am here to help you along the way. If you ever need anything, please shoot me an email. You can reach me any time at PatFlynn@ChroniclesOfStrength.com.

My story with fasting: Dr. Kellyann

I've always loved a good mystery — the challenge of figuring something out based on my observations. Growing up, I was the roving reporter. You could find me casing the neighborhood, pen and paper in hand and always ready to crack the case.

As I entered my career, my ever-present curiosity evolved from a "whodunit" to more of a "whatdunit" — specifically, what causes people's health to fail and what causes the body to look and feel its best. It's no wonder I became a health practitioner, and, to that end, it's no wonder I discovered fasting.

I learned early on in the clinic that I was really, for all intents and purposes, in the solutions business. People came to me wanting answers, and I often found them. That's how I became attracted to fasting. So many of my patients faced time crunches and roadblocks on their paths to health. I realized if I could find a diet tool that would add simplicity and not steal time, patients just might get some good results.

Channeling the detective Nancy Drew, I searched maniacally for a system that would meet those goals. What I found seemed like an oversimplification. Rather profound, really. Eat healthy, real foods, with an intentional short-term "pattern-interrupt," where you give your body a break from eating.

I realized a positive outcome could happen from what you *don't* do, rather than what you *do* do. As I myself adopted the fasting principles, I was blown away. It provided my life with flexibility and ease. I lost body fat, increased muscle mass, decreased my insulin levels, and increased growth hormones. Bottom line: I looked younger, stronger, and leaner, and I felt fantastic — without much hassle.

I knew whatever was happening was happening on a cellular level — that my body was going through some kind of "internal housekeeping." This was a strategy worth sharing.

I have since communicated the message of fasting to the masses. I believe eating healthy, real foods with an intentional short-term "pattern-interrupt" can be the solution for so many who want to look and feel their best.

For fasting news, tips, and inspiration, visit my website, www.drkellyann.com, or follow me on twitter @drkellyann.

Chapter 2

Navigating the Science of Fasting

Standard dieting in the United States often sounds like this: "Hey, you got fat by eating, so instead of eating that, eat this." Okay, so you're overweight by *eating*, and now to get thin, you want to eat. That just doesn't sound or look consistent or logical. This line of thinking seems broken. But admittedly, it works in most instances — at least for a little while. But we ask you, wouldn't it be far more sensible, and far more effective, for people who gained weight by eating to simply stop eating?

The answer, of course, is yes. And in this chapter, we explain why. We break it all down for you — both the science and philosophy behind fasting. We examine how fasting works to help you lose fat and gain muscle at the same time, how fasting can help your mind think more clearly, and how fasting can help build your body's defenses against everyday illnesses as well as major diseases. Add some intense exercise to your fasting regime and you may be surprised at the results. (We also discuss how you can eat when you're not fasting to be more healthy.)

Fasting isn't starving yourself. Starvation is a *severe* nutritional, caloric, and vitamin deficiency and is a prolonged condition. On the other hand, fasting is taking a short break from eating. The two don't even compare.

Losing Fat and Gaining Muscle

Fasting can help you lose fat and gain muscle. But we won't mislead you — losing fat and gaining muscle are two diametrically opposed goals. One requires a caloric surplus, the other a deficit. Any hype about doing both at the same time is plainly hype. After all, the law of thermodynamics states that all matter and energy is constant, which tells you that it's simply impossible to gain weight unless you take in an overconsumption of calories. It's non-negotiable. It's the law of thermodynamics. Not an idea. Not a theory. The law, sure as gravity.

What you can do, however, is lose fat while still preserving lean muscle mass. Or, on the opposite end, you can add muscle mass while maintaining your relative body fat percentage — that is, adding lean muscle mass. Fasting assists with both.

These sections look more closely at how exactly fasting helps you to build muscle more efficiently and lose fat more effortlessly.

Don't try to do everything at once. Of course you may want to build muscle and lose fat at the same time. Who wouldn't? But things don't necessarily work that way. Focus on one thing first. That is, your first goal should be to have just one goal.

Burning more body fat

When you take a break from eating, your body burns more fat. So yes, not eating — perhaps the most classically employed method of weight loss — in almost all cases, is still the safest and soundest option for weight loss.

In order to understand how fasting assists in the process of burning fat, we need to first explain how fat burning works. To burn body fat, you must get fatty acids out from hiding (out from stored body fat, that is) and into the bloodstream (a process known as *lipolysis*). You can initiate lipolysis in a couple ways:

- Exercise
- Fasting (yes, not eating)

But you're not done yet. The fatty acids must then be burnt off (a process known as *oxidation*) in the mitochondria of your muscle cells. After the fatty acids are burnt off, they're dead. Gone for good. Sayonara.

Fasting increases lipolysis through a sort of default. That is, as soon as your body is done digesting its last meal, it then begins lipolysis for sustained energy, releasing fatty acids into the bloodstream. This process may start to happen as early as two hours into a fast. The longer you fast, the more fatty acids are released into your bloodstream — up to a point, of course.

But again, releasing fat into the bloodstream isn't enough. Eating too soon may actually drive those fatty acids back into storage in a process known as *re-esterification.* To ensure that the fatty acids are burned up, you must stretch your fasting periods to various lengths, to allow the oxidation process to take place. If you really want to kill fat dead, then you ought to add exercise into the fasted state. (Refer to the "Amplifying the effects of exercise" section later in this chapter for more information.)

In 2005, the American Society for Clinical Nutrition featured a study on alternate-day fasting — which is a full fast every other day — on nonobese subjects. After 22 days, the subjects lost, on average, 2.5 percent of their body mass. What's more interesting is that they lost, on average, 4 percent of their initial fat mass.

Making muscle gain easier

Fasting along with exercise during your fasting state can also help your body put on muscle. The human body has a special protein called *mammalian target of rapamycin (mTOR* for short). Many experts now refer to it as the muscle-building gene, because recent research shows that it regulates the construction and rejuvenation of muscle tissue.

When mTOR is activated, it triggers muscle *hypertrophy* (an increase in muscle size) through an increase in protein *synthesis* (how your body turns protein into muscle tissue). Basically when mTOR is on, it helps you build muscle. But you can go overboard. If mTOR is on too much, it loses its potency, can become hyperactive, and bad things can start to happen (overactive mTOR activity has been linked to irregular cell growth and various forms of cancer).

Two things can activate mTOR:

- ✔ **The hormone insulin:** The pancreas secretes insulin. Because insulin is a blood sugar regulator, it's released whenever you eat and serves to shuttle nutrients into cells.

Too much insulin (chronically elevated levels of insulin) is a deleterious dilemma and may lead to a host of malaises, not limited to, but including

- Alzheimer's disease

- Diabetes

- Heart disease

- Insulin resistance

- Various forms of cancer

✔ **Intense exercise:** Intense exercise actually activates mTOR by first suppressing it. When you begin to exercise, mTOR is inhibited, suppressed like a spring. After you finish exercising, mTOR is super-sensitive, holding massive muscle-building potential. It's ready to be released as soon as you consume food.

In order to increase mTOR's muscle-making potential, you must first suppress it. And you suppress it by not eating. That way, when you do unleash it — either through eating, exercise, or a combination of the two — the effects are amplified.

If insulin is chronically elevated, you can grow quite insensitive to its effects — even to the point of developing diabetes. And because insulin activates mTOR, you can also lose your ability to gain muscle efficiently through chronically elevated levels of insulin.

You can call this the perpetual cycle of doom: The more you eat, the more insulin you produce and the less sensitive you become to it. The less sensitive you become to insulin, the more you need to get the same job done and the more insulin you produce. And the more insulin you produce . . . you get the point. So you can then deduce that if your aim is to build muscle, then eating more isn't the best long-term solution.

You can never turn off insulin, but you can turn it down. Fasting is one of the best ways, if not *the* best way, to balance your insulin levels. If you control your insulin levels and bring them down to a more balanced level, you can become more sensitive to its effects. That is, you'll need less insulin to get the job done, which can help you build muscle more efficiently.

In order to control your insulin levels, you can try some of the various diets available, such as the Paleo Diet and the Mediterranean Diet. (Check out Kellyann's book, *Paleo Cookbook For Dummies,* and *The Mediterranean Diet Cookbook* by Meri Raffetto and Wendy Jo Peterson, both by John Wiley & Sons, Inc., for more information.) You can also refer to the later section, "Eating Healthful Meals When You're Not Fasting" to manage your insulin when you're not fasting. And although eating healthily is very important, the best thing you can do to balance your insulin levels is to not eat at all. Once again, fasting prevails.

Improving Brain Function and Productivity

The research is clear: Fasting helps to ward off the odds of neurodegenerative diseases. In fact, even if you have no interest in losing weight or gaining muscle, the positive benefits of fasting on the brain alone merit your great consideration. In fact, fasting puts mild stresses on brain cells, similar to how exercise does on the muscles. Your brain grows stronger and more resistant to neurodegenerative diseases through fasting. These sections explain how fasting works to improve your neural circuitry, bolster concentration, and enhance focus.

A common objection to fasting is the false notion that you won't be able to concentrate when you're hungry. And although this may be true at first, all the evidence points to the contrary in the long run. Those individuals who stick it out and adapt to a fasting lifestyle often report improved attention span, concentration, and focus.

Regenerating the brain

Fasting keeps the brain healthy in more than one way. Here are just a few of the major benefits fasting has on the brain — the center of the nervous system and the very thing that separates humans from apes, monkeys, and congressmen:

- **Fasting upsurges a process known as autophagy.** Think of *autophagy* as a sort of cellular waste removal service. It disposes of damaged molecules, ones that may be tied to neurological diseases. Really, it's the brain's way of taking out the trash, and without it, the garbage piles up. Through fasting, this cellular cleansing may run its course, ensuring that the brain both develops and functions optimally.

- **Fasting increases a protein known as brain-derived neurotrophic factor (BDNF).** *BDNF* prevents stressed neurons from dying. Low levels of BDNF have been linked to Alzheimer's, dementia, and other cognitive disorders.

✔ **Fasting also spurs the growth of new brain cells.** This process, known as *neurogenesis,* helps to establish new connections in the brain and may very well improve your cognitive abilities.

The brain follows the same "use it or lose it" principle that muscles do. If you want to keep your brain strong and healthy, you have to stress it from time to time. Fasting (along with physical exercise and mental exercises) can help you.

Increasing your productivity

Food is a distraction. So imagine now, briefly, how much time you would save and how much more work you would get done if you didn't have to eat. Fasting allows you to focus. It sets your mind on a smooth and steady course, so to speak. You don't have to worry about what's for breakfast, or where you're going to get lunch. Those concerns become obsolete — at least on your fasting days.

Some scientific circles believe that during the morning and for most of the daytime, people are meant to be on the move, expending energy (hunting and gathering, if you will). Only when night comes along are people meant to eat, relax, and recuperate. Some say this is the natural order of things, or a human's natural biorhythm. We discuss this philosophy more when we explain the Warrior Diet in Chapter 7.

After you discover how to get in tune with your hunger, which may take a couple of days or even a few weeks, you can find that concentration comes easy, in fact easier than it probably ever did before. Some scientists believe this concentration factor is linked to a sort of primal mechanism. That is, hunger provides impetus to get work done, which makes sense, because hunger compels one to hunt and to scavenge. Hunger clearly requires focus.

Think about it another way. What do you want to do after a big lunch? You probably want to take a big nap. After you eat, your body releases certain hormones that quite often make you feel sleepy. Surely you know that feeling. And you should also note that digestion itself requires much energy that you could otherwise direct toward more productive endeavors.

Hunger can be a distraction as well, but through fasting, you can train yourself to embrace hunger and discover how to use it to your advantage. Check out Chapter 14 for ways to manage your hunger and stay focused.

Boosting Your Immunity to Live Longer

Individuals who engage in calorie restriction tend to live longer. In fact, many cultures that regularly engage in such practices have shown to extend their lives.

However long-term calorie restriction does have its downsides. Aside from the general bummer of just not being able to eat as much, here are a few of the other problems that may follow chronic calorie restriction:

- ✔ Calorie counting (boring)
- ✔ Decreased energy levels
- ✔ Hunger pangs
- ✔ Loss of muscle mass
- ✔ Reduced bone mineral density

The good news is that you may not have to suffer through them to achieve a longer life. Recent research and empirical evidence suggests that fasting may produce the same longevity boosting effects that calorie restriction does, but without any of those pesky side effects.

In the following sections, we review how fasting may help you to live longer and be free from ailments as far as practicable. What you can discover is that not eating does indeed produce all the same benefits of calorie restriction, and then some.

Extending your life expectancy

Fasting has shown to increase cellular stress response, which is impaired with age. Aging is cellular degradation; it's quite simply a loss of function. *Free radicals,* which are toxic byproducts of metabolism, latch on to and destroy healthy cells and cause aging.

The moment that you're born, the second law of thermodynamics, also known as the *universal forces of entropy,* which degrades all living things, begins to attack you. It's just what it is, and you can't do anything to change that. You can, however, choose to not accept death so easily. You do in fact have the equipment to defend yourself. This natural arsenal of weaponry to combat aging includes all the natural rejuvenation processes to fight off oxidative damage, such as the *antioxidant system* (any collection of enzymes that serve as a person's natural cellular defense mechanisms). And guess what can help you use it to the fullest possible extent. You guessed it. Fasting is one of the two ways to combat premature aging (the other being exercise).

It's no wonder nature favors the lean and wiry. Fasting is an acute stressor, much like exercise, and through stressors, your body can thrive. In fact, hunger and exercise are specifically the primal rejuvenation triggers. Studies have shown, again and again, that the human body flourishes when faced with physical and nutritional challenges. In fact, a 1982 study found that mice fed every other day outlived mice fed regularly by 82 percent. This rejuvenation happens through the process of autophagy (refer to the earlier section, "Regenerating the brain" for more information).

Furthermore, eating, especially heavy eating, actually hastens the aging process. Too much insulin and mTOR overactivity speed up the rate of cellular degradation. And so, as you may expect, people combat aging by not eating.

Here are some of the positive physiological benefits brought about from a lack of food:

✔ Cellular cleansing and tissue rejuvenation

✔ Improved body composition

✔ Increased energy efficiency

✔ Increased resistance to fatigue

Physical hardship, or *stress,* isn't what kills people. Pleasures are what kill people. Overindulgence is what kills people. Through stress, people thrive, and hardship makes the body grow stronger. In other words, those people who eat less tend to live longer. But there's more to it than that. People who eat less also tend to live healthier.

Warding off disease

Fasting may not only help you live longer, but be healthier as well. It's very difficult to live long if you're relatively unhealthy, so fasting also makes sense to ward off illness. As a matter of fact, fasting is perhaps the world's oldest cure-all and the most potent natural remedy for whatever ails you. Everyone actually has a natural inclination to resist food when they're ill. These sections specifically identify two main ways that fasting can help you fend off disease.

Fasting restores proper pH balance in the blood. When the body's pH balance gets out of whack, misery is certain. Too much acidity in the blood can lead to *acidosis*, which often leads to many debilitating ailments like arthritis. Fasting works to clear acidosis from the bloodstream and to restore the proper alkaline-acidity environment needed for the body to thrive.

None of this discussion on fasting stuff is new. Upton Sinclair wrote a book called *The Fasting Cure* in 1911, and, at the time, it was a bestseller. The only difference from then and now: People have the technology and the science to validate what has always been know — fasting is very good for you.

Keeping insulin levels in check

Fasting helps to ward off the odds of disease by fixing the root problem of almost all diseases — too much insulin brought about by too much food. Fasting controls insulin levels, and, in turn, improves insulin sensitivity. And you also know that unchecked insulin levels lead to insulin resistance. Here are just a few diseases linked to insulin resistance:

- ✔ Breast cancer
- ✔ Diabetes
- ✔ Heart attack
- ✔ Metabolic syndrome
- ✔ Prostate cancer

So you can reasonably assume that any measured aim at controlling insulin levels is a measured aim at combatting disease.

Decreasing chronic inflammation

Fasting also helps to reduce chronic inflammation, which many doctors say is the true number-one killer in the United States. In fact, fasting, as well as calorie restriction with a healthy, low-glycemic diet, such as the Paleo Diet or Mediterranean Diet, can control chronic inflammation.

Inflammation is the body's natural response to any harmful stimuli, ranging from a bacterial infection to a bump on the head. Inflammation not only serves as a *protective-casting mechanism* (such as when you stub your toe and the toe reddens), so that you don't reinjure yourself, but also has the job of hunting down pathogens and breaking down tissue.

When it comes to eating, everything you put into your body matters. It either serves to better you or injure you. Your health is largely the accumulation of all the food decisions you've ever made.

Inflammation can be either acute or chronic.

Dealing with illness and injury: Acute inflammation

Acute, or short-lived, inflammation is necessary to handle and correct injury and illness. Here are a few instances that can bring about acute inflammation:

- ✔ Allergies and other irritants
- ✔ Bacterial or viral infection
- ✔ Burns or frostbite
- ✔ Cuts, scrapes, and lacerations
- ✔ Physical injuries (falling off a bike, stubbing your toe, and so on)

And here are the classic signs of acute inflammation:

- ✔ Inhibited or loss of function
- ✔ Pain/tenderness
- ✔ Redness
- ✔ Swelling

Lasting long-term: Chronic inflammation

The problem though is more with chronic inflammation where the inflammation doesn't turn off, but instead becomes a constant low-level and systemic occurrence. Chronic inflammation is when your own defense mechanism turns against you.

Here are some of the diseases linked to chronic inflammation:

- ✔ Arthritis
- ✔ Cardiovascular disease
- ✔ Diabetes
- ✔ Fatty liver
- ✔ Hypertension
- ✔ Metabolic syndrome
- ✔ Various forms of cancer

Inflammation obviously is a complicated matter and one that scientists don't fully understand. But as more and more evidence emerges, it's becoming abundantly clear that chronic inflammation plays a very significant role in the progression of illness and disease.

And you probably aren't surprised to hear that chronic inflammation is closely tied to overeating and obesity. Once again unchecked insulin levels are largely to blame. Here are some of the other causes of inflammation:

- ✔ Poor food choices, including eating too much and eating low-quality and toxic foods
- ✔ High amounts of stress
- ✔ Lack of sleep
- ✔ Lack of exercise/movement

As you can see, most of the causes of chronic inflammation are prolonged activities in and of themselves. What really brings about chronic inflammation is a prolonged series of poor decisions that a person makes.

Focusing on Your Energy Level and Exercise

Fasting, at first, can be draining. And we don't want you to think that everything with fasting is rainbows and unicorns. Compare it to the first time you worked out intensely after some time in between workouts. More than likely, you were exhausted, right? But if you stuck with it, surely you found it became easier and easier.

Fasting works much the same way. It's a difficult stress to endure, but only at first. After you're conditioned to the fasted state or adapted to a fasting lifestyle, fasting becomes no more strenuous an activity than brisk walking is for the conditioned runner.

These sections examine how fasting serves to boost energy levels and amplify the positive effects of exercise. Contrary to popular belief, fasting doesn't bog you down, nor impair your ability to work out intensely, quite the opposite, actually!

If at any time during your fast you feel excessively lightheaded or unable to function, have a small snack. Adapting to the fasted time takes time, and it even takes more time to function optimally while fasted. Ease your way into it and don't push too far too fast.

Increasing your energy

Fasting actually works to increase your energy in a similar way that exercise does. The body responds to stress via the release of *adrenaline,* a person's natural *fight-or-flight hormone.* Typically, the bigger the stress you experience, the bigger the adrenal response is. For example, if a lion were chasing you or you were being held at gunpoint, you would experience a massive adrenaline surge, which is your natural response to danger.

When your adrenal glands release adrenaline and noradrenaline, you feel awake, alert, and ready for action. When your body enters a fight-or-flight mode, your body goes into survival mode and you typically experience the following physiological processes:

- Accelerated breathing
- Constriction of blood vessels
- Increased heart rate
- Liberation of energy stores (fat and glycogen) into the bloodstream
- Pupil dilation
- Tunnel vision

Fasting isn't such a large stressor, though, so the adrenaline response is far milder, but it's still enough to provide a natural boost in adrenaline. The adrenal response to fasting also helps to explain why fasting is so darn effective for fat loss, because adrenaline helps to drive energy stores, such as fat and muscle glycogen, out of storage and into the bloodstream to maintain energy output and blood sugar. You can almost think of adrenaline as the key that unlocks stored body fat. Refer to the earlier section, "Burning more body fat" for additional information.

Furthermore, this extra adrenaline explains how fasting boosts energy, focus, and concentration, rather than inhibiting them. With fasting, all the hormones are in healthy balance. Too much adrenaline, like too much anything, is a bad thing. But you don't have to worry about having too much adrenaline from the occasional fast, especially not in a society where most people already abuse their adrenals with the overuse of stimulants. For specific suggestions on how you can boost your energy when you're fasting, check out Chapter 16.

Amplifying the effects of exercise

The combination of fasting and exercise triggers an amazing rejuvenation and detoxification process, far beyond what exercise and fasting offer by themselves. In other words, fasting and exercise, when joined, enhance the benefits of one another.

You can assume that all the benefits to be had from exercising are increased when you exercise in a fasted state, such as an increase in the following:

✔ Cellular stress response (to protect us against illness and aging)

✔ Fat burning (lipolysis)

✔ Insulin sensitivity (making it easier to build more lean muscle)

✔ Muscle tissue repair

✔ *Neurogenesis* (the birth of new brain cells)

The reverse is also true, meaning that the benefits to be had from fasting are increased when you add in exercise. You can look at it from either angle. The body responds to negatives positively. Hardship in the form of fasting and exercise is a trigger for growth. Without adversity, prowess fades away.

And so you may be wondering, what is the best way you can combine fasting and exercise? It largely depends on what sort of fasting protocol you choose to follow. We cover the pros and cons of the most popular fasting methods today in the chapters in Part II, but for now, just know that exercise is best added toward the end of your fasting period because exercise in a fasted state plows fertile ground for muscle growth and rejuvenation. You can also check out Chapter 11 that provides more insight into the effects of combining exercise and fasting.

To really kick-start the muscle-building process, you need to eat within the window of opportunity, the 30 to 60 minutes after your workout, which is when your muscles are most receptive to nutrients and will most effectively utilize these nutrients to build and rejuvenate muscle tissue. In other words, when your muscles are hungry, they have priority. During this window, you should have your largest meal, because the fuel you take in, so long as you don't overdo it, will go toward replenishing muscle glycogen and repairing muscle tissue, instead of being stored as body fat.

All these benefits we discuss here come from short and intense bouts of exercise, such as heavy strength training, power training, speed training, or metabolic conditioning. For more on high-intensity exercise and a full 90-day body transformation program, please check out our other book *Paleo Workouts For Dummies* (John Wiley & Sons, Inc.).

Debunking Common Fasting Myths

We wish we could just tell you that everything you've probably ever heard about fasting is wrong and leave it at that. Instead, we want to give you what you'll need to defend your fasting practices against those naysayers who still suffer from conventional wisdom — that is, those who still believe in fairy tales.

Whatever information you've heard or been told that says fasting is bad for you is either wholly unsupported or very plainly wrong. These sections analyze these myths and break them down so you can fast with peace of mind and defend your actions against all those individuals who may question them.

Slowing your metabolism

This myth is a classic, and how the foolish idea that your metabolism, if not fueled every couple of hours, will slow down became so widely accepted is beyond us. Your *metabolism* is the energy cost to keep your cells alive; it's the summation of all the biological processes that sustain your life. For the most part, your basal metabolic rate is tied closely to your weight.

No matter where this myth came from, it's simply not true, because despite popular belief, researchers have proven many times over that only the *amount* of food you eat matters, not the *pattern* in which you eat it. That's to say, how frequently you eat or when you eat doesn't dictate your body composition. The only thing that matters and the only thing that has ever mattered is how much you eat in terms of weight and body composition. In terms of health, the *quality* of what you eat matters very much as well.

To take a closer look at this myth, we look at the false idea that your metabolism has different speeds, or that it is something that can be sped up or slowed down. Your metabolism is the collection of all the entire biological processes that sustain life. It's not some mystical fire in your gut. And it's not something that you should be trying to constantly speed up. Rather it's something you should be trying to optimize.

Fasting doesn't decrease your metabolism, nor does it put you into starvation mode. Starvation mode is a myth, unless of course, you're actually suffering from starvation, which then it's very real. But you're not starving with fasting, not even close.

The truth is, you're going to burn whatever amount of calories you're going to burn. Aside from adding in exercise, there's really no other way to burn more calories. The only way to lose weight is to eat less, move more, or both.

Eating more frequently isn't the solution. It never was. Eating all the time improves your metabolism to the very same extent that keeping your eyes always open improves your eyesight, which is to say not at all. In fact, fasting gives your digestive system a chance to rest, like blinking does for the eyes.

When you stop to think about it, eating more frequently doesn't make any sense from a weight-loss perspective. For example, say it takes 20 calories to digest 200 calories, which is about accurate. Now who, wanting to burn 20 calories, in their right mind, would ever eat 200 calories to do so? It's just a ludicrous idea and completely broken logic! But really, it's what this whole "speed up your metabolism" thing is based around.

You may have known some people who eat frequently and who still lose weight. Frequent feeding diets still work, as long as they put someone in a calorie deficit. The only problem, however, is that over time too much frequent feeding may lead to decreased insulin sensitivity and other health problems. Refer to the earlier section, "Making muscle gain easier" for more about these potential health problems.

Gaining the weight back after eating

Some people claim that fasting, or dieting in general, is a waste of time because you'll simply just gain the weight back after you stop. That's why we say that fasting is a lifestyle change. It's not a diet. It's a permanent fixture.

If your goal is to lose weight, then the reason you're thinking of or have already started fasting is because you were consuming more calories than you were expending, and you needed to reverse it. If you stop fasting, and so reverse it again, of course you'll gain back the weight, because you went right back to taking in more calories than you were putting out. You can't just go back to your old ways and think everything's going to be different because you spent a few weeks on a diet. If you do what you've always done, then you're going to get exactly what you've always had. This is why we say quite deliberately that fasting is a lifestyle change. It's not a diet. It's a permanent fixture.

A lifestyle change means that you form a new and permanent series of habits. In other words, you follow a new order of daily operations. You think differently. You act differently. You eat differently. This is how you produce change. And, more importantly, this is how you sustain change.

A common misconception entangled in this myth is that you'll immediately gain back the weight after you stop fasting. That idea is true only if you overcompensate, by taking in additional calories to make up for those lost during your fast.

We clearly don't recommend you do that because you fasted in the first place to lose weight and assume a caloric deficit, and the only way to reduce surplus weight is to assume a calorie deficit. Eating after a fast shouldn't be a binge. Read the later section, "Eating Healthful Meals When You're Not Fasting" to find out what to eat when you go off a fast.

Other people may say that the weight you lose fasting is simply the loss of water weight or muscle glycogen. Although that may be true in some cases, it's far from the whole truth. The truth is that you will lose weight in the form of body fat. It won't be immediate, but, if you stick with your fasting protocol, it will be a sure thing.

Fat loss is a slow, dripping process. Anyone can cut water weight quickly. Fasting isn't a means to reduce water weight. As a matter of fact, in Chapter 13, we emphasize the importance of drinking plenty of water while fasting.

Having lower energy without food

At first, you may experience a few complaints while fasting, one of which may be decreased energy. (Chapter 3 mentions a few other complaints you may have when you first start to fast and how to set a positive mindset to deal with them.) After your body and mind adapt to the fasting lifestyle, you won't even think twice about having less energy when skipping meals. You'll feel vibrant and vigorous. You'll have the energy of a thousand suns.

Refer to the earlier section, "Focusing on Your Energy Level and Exercise" for more information about how fasting works to boost energy through increased adrenaline. You can also think of this: Hunger is a motivator, perhaps the most primal motivator of all. Predators hunt when they're hungry. When they're hungry, they expend the most energy. Think of fasting as being on the hunt, as a time when your body is primed to get its most taxing work done.

But at the same time try to not focus too much on the hunger. Keep yourself busy. Actually, when starting out, fast on a day that you know you're going to be busy. Keeping yourself distracted and on the go makes fasting a more tolerable and pleasant experience.

Eating Healthy When You're Not Fasting

Even though fasting may reduce the effects of poor eating habits, it's not a powerful enough mechanism to completely prevent or reverse the ailments brought about from an unhealthy diet. What you eat when not fasting is just as important as the practice of fasting itself. Without proper nutrition, the benefits of fasting are severely inhibited.

Fasting alone isn't enough to save you from all the negative effects of poor nutrition. Not eating is a healthy activity, and the only way you can make not eating unhealthy is if you overdo it. Eating, on the other hand, can either be a healthy activity or a not-so-healthy activity.

You must realize that everything you put into your body either serves to improve your health or degrades it. There is no gray area — certain foods promote vibrant health at the cellular level, whereas other foods seek to destroy it.

These sections can help you to understand the importance of quality food selection and a natural, whole foods–based diet. We discuss the importance of controlling blood sugar and the role of the glycemic index. And lastly we dive into the details of what we believe to be the perfect complement to fasting: the Paleo Diet.

Understanding the glycemic index

The best approach to eating is a low-glycemic diet, and one that is centered on wholesome, nutritious foods. A *low-glycemic diet is* any diet aimed at controlling blood sugar. When considering a low-glycemic diet, make sure you consider these two factors:

- ✔ **Glycemic index:** The *glycemic index* tells you how quickly your blood sugar rises after eating a certain food. Foods that have a high glycemic index, such as sugary foods, tend to spike insulin levels and raise blood sugar very quickly.

- ✔ **Glycemic load:** The *glycemic load* tells you how much a food spikes your insulin and raises your blood sugar overall, regardless of time. Typically, the more carbs a food contains, the higher the glycemic load, but not necessarily the glycemic index. For example, whole grains, because they're digested slowly, typically have a lower glycemic index, but because they're carb heavy, they tend to have a higher glycemic load.

So, if you want to eat for health and leanness, then your aim must be to focus your diet around foods that are low glycemic — that is, foods that have both a low glycemic index and low glycemic load. These foods include lean protein sources (such as chicken and turkey), fatty protein sources (such as a grass-fed steak), healthy fat sources (such as nuts, seeds, or extra-virgin olive oil), most vegetables (such as broccoli, cauliflower, and so on), and some fruits (such as blueberries and blackberries).

Eating like a caveman

When you're not fasting, we suggest you follow the Paleo Diet, which is also known as the *Caveman Diet*. This method of eating aims to replicate the eating habits of your ancestors. In short, when you're on this diet, you eat the foods you're biologically designed to eat.

When we say biologically designed, we mean that from a genetic composition standpoint, humans have changed very little over the past 40,000 years. The advent of agriculture, which is a relatively recent invention in the grand scheme of things (relatively recent as in the last 10,000 years) hasn't significantly influenced our genes, which is also true of the Industrial Revolution. Hence, humans simply aren't adapted to eat many of the foods that the agricultural and industrial revolutions have made so readily available — namely, grains and processed foods. Many physicians, nutritionists, scientists, and anthropologists believe that the poor dietary habits established since the dawn of the agricultural and industrial revolutions are the root causes of illnesses such as heart disease, cancer, diabetes, and hypertension.

The flip side is that scientists now also understand that a blueprint for optimal nutrition resides in all humans' genes. This blueprint, which is a set of rules for what humans are designed to eat, was distilled by looking at how our ancestors used to eat, specifically our Paleolithic ancestors. And this blueprint is what many nutritionists call the Paleo Diet, or the Caveman Diet.

Just like fasting, the Paleo Diet has you call in question many commonly held beliefs, such as the idea that whole grains are a necessary part of a balanced diet. This idea, of course, would be false. Whole grains are by no means necessary. In fact, you can find anything that is beneficial in whole grains elsewhere for fewer calories and fewer carbohydrates. These sections provide more insight into the Paleo Diet. If you're interested in making a lifestyle change to this diet, check out *Living Paleo For Dummies* by Melissa Joulwan and me (Kellyann) and my (Kellyann) book, *Paleo Cookbook For Dummies,* both by John Wiley & Sons, Inc.

Helping you lose weight

Not only does the Paleo Diet promote a sustainable and sound approach to nutrition, but it also helps with the weight loss process as well, and here's why:

  ✔ **You eat nutrient-dense foods.** *Nutrient-dense* means foods that pack the most nutrition (such as vitamins, minerals, antioxidants, and amino acids) in the least amount of calories. You want to consume foods that your body can actually use, such as lean protein, fibrous vegetables, and healthy fats, while avoiding junk calories, which means no candy, no breads, and no soft drinks.

✓ **You eat low-glycemic foods.** Doing so can help you maintain healthy blood sugar and insulin levels, shifting your body's preferred fuel source from sugar to fat (this is what many refer to as being *fat-adapted*).

Furthermore, because the Paleo Diet balances out blood sugar, you'll have increased energy for more effective workout sessions.

✓ **You eat healthier and feel fuller.** Because of an emphasis on healthy fats, protein, and leafy vegetables, you're fuller for longer than you otherwise would on a higher carb diet, consuming less calories overall.

Putting together your meals

These lists are by no means all-inclusive, but they can give you a good idea of where to start, and provide you with everything you need to organize a healthy, balanced, Paleolithic meal. Before we dive in directly, here are a few basic guidelines when it comes to constructing your meals:

✓ **Consume protein at every meal.** Protein has the highest thermic effect of food (meaning it takes more calories for the body to process protein than it does carbohydrates or fats) and promotes a greater sense of *satiety* (fullness) than carbohydrates do.

✓ **Always consume a source of fibrous vegetables at each meal.** Examples include broccoli, asparagus, and cauliflower. Vegetables such as these pack tons of nutrients in very few calories and will further promote satiety.

✓ **Eat starchy carbohydrates last.** Starchy carbohydrates such as sweet potatoes are denser in terms of calories and carbohydrates than vegetables of the leafy variety. This isn't to say that they should be avoided entirely, only consumed judiciously. As a general rule, if you're going to have starchy carbohydrates, consume them last — after proteins, vegetables, and healthy fats — when you're less hungry and therefore less likely to overdo it.

✓ **Eat to satisfaction not to fullness.** That is, take your time eating your meals and enjoy the food. Don't shovel it down for the sake of shoveling it down.

Defending the Paleo Diet

Some anthropologists have debated on whether or not cavemen (people from the Paleolithic era) really ate Paleo, but that discussion really is of no concern today, because here' s the thing: Good eating should be concise. Just as a sentence should contain no unnecessary words, a meal should contain no unnecessary foods, and a diet no unnecessary meals. The Paleo Diet works because it helps you to focus on what is necessary and to weed out what is unnecessary.

The secret to a good diet is to strip it down to the fundamentals — powerful proteins, healthy fats, fibrous vegetables, nutrient-dense fruits — and to leave it at that. A good diet is clean, tidy, and organized, and has in it only the essentials. A bad diet is a teenager's bedroom.

Additionally, the Paleo Diet is reasonable. It isn't about deprivation; you can sustain it long-term. Furthermore, the hormone-balancing, anti-inflammatory, and nutrient-dense qualities of the Paleo Diet work toward combating the following ailments:

- Aches and pains
- Autoimmune problems
- Cardiovascular disease
- Depression
- Diabetes

- Digestive issues
- Fatigue
- Menstrual problems
- Skin issues
- Weight gain

The Paleo Diet is the perfect complement to fasting. Together, fasting and the Paleo Diet are the evolutionary keys to unlocking true health, leanness, and vitality.

Tracking Your Health Progress

Although we're hesitant to call fasting a traditional diet (think of fasting more as just a regular part of your lifestyle), when starting out on any new exercise or nutrition regimen, the best way to see what kind of progress you're making is to benchmark certain variables, such as your total weight, body fat levels, and routine blood tests.

This way, after adhering to whichever fasting protocol that you're trying, you can easily track your progress. Seeing the progress you've made is much harder if you're only going by what you see in the mirror each day. If you don't track certain measurements — and which measurements you do track is completely up to you — you run the risk of losing sight of your goals and losing motivation. If you don't know where exactly you've started, then seeing see all the wonderful gains you're making via fasting is difficult.

Here are some ways that you can better gauge the process that you're making while fasting.

Weighing yourself

One way that people track their progress is by weighing themselves on their bathroom scales. However, we urge you not to trust your scales as a reflection of your progress.

Although you may think that stepping on a scale is the easiest way to track your progress, we disagree. People get too hung up on what the number on the scale reads, and the scale, by nature, only tells a part of the story. It only tells you your total body weight, not a breakdown of what your fat-to-muscle ratio is. Many people who begin a healthy lifestyle overhaul will notice that at times, their total body weight actually goes up because lean muscle mass is dense and weighs more than body fat. You want to have more lean muscle mass on your body, but your typical bathroom scale isn't going to be able to show you that. As a result, don't rely solely on your total weight as an indicator of success.

Testing your body fat

You can get a better picture of not only your body weight, but also your body-fat composition by measuring you body-fat composition in a couple different ways. However, these methods are also notoriously inaccurate.

- **Body-fat composition scales:** Some scales can measure your body weight and your overall body-fat composition. A seemingly endless array of factors contribute to the accuracy of the results, anything from how hydrated you are to whether you have calloused or dirty feet. A 2008 study found that body composition scales underestimated the body-fat percentages of overweight and obese people and overestimated the percentages of leaner people. Even the user manuals for these devices say that they may not be very accurate for athletes, the elderly, children, people with osteoporosis, and so on. (Some hand-held body composition scales have been shown to be slightly more accurate but not completely so.)

- **Body-fat calipers:** You can find someone, such as a personal trainer or physician, who is experienced in using body-fat calipers to measure your body fat. *Body-fat calipers* pinch the fat on your body in several key points, including the triceps, hips, and bellybutton areas. These measurements are then plugged into an equation that can give you your body-fat percentage. However, this method can also be inaccurate because you need someone's help who knows how to use the calipers, and even then, human error is quite high.

Body composition scales and calipers *are* good at one thing: trending. So even if the numbers they give aren't incredibly accurate, they will go down — or up — according to your adherence to your fast and exercise program. Being able to see these numbers and how they change over time can serve to help keep you motivated and on track.

✔ **Water displacement or air displacement test:** If you want a very accurate picture of your body composition, you can consider scheduling a water displacement or air displacement test, such as a Bod Pod test. However, you may find that one of these tests isn't within your budget (they typically cost $50 or more for a single test). Furthermore, they may not be wholly necessary for you and your goals. Cheaper options are available for tracking your progress, which we discuss in the "Considering other benchmarks" section.

No matter what method you use (if you use any), make sure you keep a log of your measurements to check the changes. If you continue fasting, you'll be able to at least see the downward trend every few months. For most people, just seeing that trend is enough. You don't need to be overly consumed with your exact numbers.

Calculating your body mass index (BMI)

Another way to keep an eye on your progress is to find out your body mass index (BMI). You calculate your BMI by looking at your height-to-weight ratio. Your BMI won't tell you your fat-to-lean mass ratio or how much body fat you have, but it will tell you if you're overweight or obese and how far into those unhealthy ranges you are.

To calculate your BMI, do the following:

1. **Weigh yourself and measure your height.**

2. **Use an online BMI calculator (which you can find using a search engine) or you can calculate manually your BMI.**

   To manually calculate your BMI, stick to these steps:

   1. **Convert your weight from pounds to kilograms by dividing your weight in pounds by 2.2 kilograms.**

      For example, 150 pounds divided by 2.2 equals 68 kilograms

   2. **Convert your height from inches to meters by dividing your height in inches by 39.37.**

      For example, 70 inches divided by 39.37 equals 1.78 meters

   3. **Calculate your BMI.**

Your weight (in kilograms) divided by your height (in meters) × your height (in meters) = BMI. For example, 68 kilograms divided by (1.78 meters × 1.78 meters) = 21.46.

Table 2-1 shows the standard BMI ranges.

Table 2-1	The BMI Ranges
BMI	*Weight Status*
Below 18.5	Underweight
18.5–24.9	Normal
25.0–29.9	Overweight
30.0 and above	Obese

A criticism of BMI is that, because it can't show body composition, if you have a lot of muscle of on your body (which weighs more than fat), you may get skewed results. However, as with the body composition or regular body weight scales, tracking your BMI may work for you simply because it's a simple, inexpensive way to see the trending of your weight loss as you begin incorporating fasting into your life and throughout your weigh-loss journey.

Taking selfies: Grab your camera

The easiest way to benchmark your starting point — and to see your progress — is to grab your camera (in these days, your camera phone) and take some self photos (that's a *selfie* for anyone older than 50). Make sure the photos show your entire body from the front, sides, and back. Because you won't have to share these photos with anyone and you'll want to see the most detail possible when you compare your before-and-after shots, wear a bathing suit or your birthday suit.

After you take them, stash them away (in a hidden folder on your computer or phone) so that you won't be tempted to look at them until after 90 days. After 90 days, you take new photos in the same conditions and compare the before-and-after photos. Photos don't lie. If you've adhered to a fasting method during those 90 days, you'll be shocked at the changes you see.

Along with your photos, you may also consider taking measurements with a soft measuring tape of your waist, hips, thighs, arms, and, for women, bust. These measurements are also quite simple to take and don't require the help of another person who is experienced in using body-fat calipers. You can then compare the before-and-after measurements to gauge your progress.

Considering other benchmarks

If you want to track other factors to mark your progress, you can consider getting routine blood work checked prior to your start of your fast and again after 90 days. All these tests are routine and inexpensive, and are typically ordered during annual visits to the doctor. These tests can include the following:

✔ **HDL and LDL cholesterol levels:** Cholesterol is broken into two types:

   • **High-density lipoprotein (HDL):** It's the good cholesterol that travels the bloodstream, looking for bad cholesterol to remove. High levels of HDL reduce your risk of heart disease.

   • **Low-density lipoprotein (LDL):** It's the bad cholesterol, collecting on the walls of blood vessels, increasing the risk of heart disease and stroke.

You're looking for a favorable ratio of the two with low LDL and high HDL.

You can improve your cholesterol ratio by fasting, as well as by consuming more foods such as walnuts, avocados, fish oil, and other healthy fats that have been shown to raise the body's HDL levels, and consuming fewer processed foods (breakfast cereal, energy bars, processed meats, breads, and other prepackaged foods) and foods containing trans fats (junk foods such as commercially prepared baked goods — cakes, cookies, donuts, and some snack foods, such as potato chips fried in shortening) that are known to increase LDL levels.

✔ **Triglycerides:** *Triglycerides* are a type of fat found in your blood that becomes stored as body fat when you burn fewer calories than you consume. Higher amounts of triglycerides increase your chances of developing heart disease. The American Heart Association states that a triglyceride level of 100 milligrams per deciliter or lower is optimal for improved heart health.

✔ **Fasting blood glucose:** This test measures how much glucose is in your blood after not eating for eight hours. Although your blood glucose levels naturally rise after you eat (we discuss the glycemic index earlier in this chapter in the "Understanding the glycemic index" section), if they stay elevated even after you've fasted, you may have diabetes or be prediabetic. Blood glucose levels that remain elevated over a long period of time can cause damage to your body in a variety of ways, including damage to your kidneys, pancreas, eyes, and nerves.

Chapter 3

Tapping Into a Successful Fasting Mindset

*M*indset is everything and everything is mindset. That is, with the proper *mindset,* In other words, your mental attitude and how you view changing your lifestyle and diet, even the worst diet, can produce impressive results. But without the proper mindset, even the best diet will fail to produce anything.

Many diets work as well as they do in the short term, because people are excited to do them. They go in with a positive and optimistic outlook, and so, they adhere to them, at least for a little while anyway. Then things get tough or boring and their outlook changes. Ultimately, their mindset changes too, and the diet and lifestyle changes fail as a result.

This chapter helps you set realistic expectations and explains how you can install a successful mindset. We purposefully say install because your mindset is programmable. You have the ability to change your mindset and outlook on life through conscious thinking. What you choose to think over time becomes your reality.

You may consider overlooking this chapter, thinking it's not important because you already have a successful mindset. Doing so wouldn't be smart. This chapter is a must read for anyone wanting to make a dietary and lifestyle change. It's the foundation from which your success will be built.

Determining Whether Fasting Is Right For You

The first question to ask yourself is whether or not fasting is right for you. Fasting isn't right for everyone, although it is right for most people.

To figure out whether fasting is right for you, ask yourself some basic questions:

- ✔ Do you want to be healthier?
- ✔ Do you want to be leaner and more energetic?
- ✔ Do you want a sustainable and reasonable approach to being healthier, leaner, and more energetic?

If your answer is yes to these questions, which we hope it is, then fasting may be right for you.

Fasting takes discipline. Nothing good comes easily, but for your disciplined efforts, fasting rewards you. Although we truly believe that fasting can work for anyone, we want to be sure that if you choose to fast, you do so from an informed position. So, in these sections, we quickly highlight the pros and cons of fasting, just so you know what you're getting yourself into, as well as how you can establish some goals to keep you on track.

The benefits of fasting reach far beyond weight loss. So even if you don't need to lose any weight, more than likely you'll still benefit from fasting in many other ways. For example, fasting can help you to put on more lean muscle mass, improve concentration, and resolve digestive issues.

Eyeing the pros and cons of fasting

Fasting, like all dietary and lifestyle practices, has its pros and cons. What's unique about fasting, however, is that many of the cons turn to pros after you shift your perspective. For example, being hungry is only a con if you make it so. You can make being hungry a positive and productive experience just by a simple shift in your mindset.

Some of the pros of fasting include the following:

- ✔ **Boosted immunity:** Fasting naturally boosts immunity and heals conditions. It's the world's oldest form of medicine, after all.

✔ **Convenient and cheaper lifestyle:** What's great about not eating for a while is that it's free.

✔ **Improved concentration:** As your energy levels increase and as you gain control over your hunger, you'll in turn find it easier to concentrate throughout the day on the most technically demanding tasks.

✔ **Increased energy:** Fasting naturally boosts energy and will help you to feel more alert and focused throughout the day.

✔ **A leaner, harder physique:** Fasting kills body fat dead. It's violent.

✔ **Sustainable long term:** Fasting isn't a quick fix. It's a lifestyle change. You can and should practice it long-term (like for the rest of your life).

✔ **Vibrant health:** You'll look and feel healthier on both the inside and out.

Note that all the benefits of fasting come as a drip, not a downpour, which is particularly true of fat loss, especially for those individuals who are already relatively lean. Fat loss is a slow and oftentimes tedious process. But with fasting, you can be sure of the process. It's going to happen; you just need to be a little patient.

Meanwhile, some of the cons typically associated with fasting include the following:

✔ **A feeling of hunger:** You will get hungry when fasting. It's unavoidable.

✔ **Occasional lightheadedness:** Getting used to being in a fasted state takes some time. And as you adapt, you may experience some uncomfortable symptoms, such as lightheadedness. They aren't dangerous, merely nuisances that will go away as your body adjusts.

✔ **Lower energy:** Along with lightheadedness, you may experience a short-term drop in energy when first embarking on your fasting journey. But it typically dissipates within one to two weeks.

✔ **The desire to binge after fasting:** The desire to binge is the biggest problem people face with fasting. To negate this con, you can start with shorter fasting periods first and gradually extend them as you become more experienced and in tune with your body.

✔ **Quite difficult in the short term:** Just like exercising for the first time in a long time isn't easy, fasting can be difficult. But after you get into the routine of it, you will feel awkward when you don't fast, just as an avid exerciser feels when not exercising.

These cons are normal occurrences that you'll encounter as you adopt a fasting lifestyle. Most of them subside after a couple of days because the initial pains of fasting are just that — initial, not permanent. Think of them as the dying of bad habits, or a sort of withdrawal period, if you will. In almost all cases, they completely reverse after you're fully acclimated to fasting. For instance, lightheadedness will typically resolve itself after the first week or two, as will the initial energy decline.

Not too bad, right? These cons are a very small price to pay for all the amazing benefits of fasting. You can see that the pros outweigh the cons by a considerable load.

We're advocating fasting for normal, healthy individuals. If you have a health or medical condition, such as diabetes, you must consult with your doctor before you embark on any type of dietary and lifestyle change such as fasting.

Setting realistic expectations and goals

In order to install a successful mindset before you begin any dietary or lifestyle change, you need to set realistic expectations for yourself to ensure both motivation and adherence. If you enter into fasting with unrealistic or downright delusional expectations, and you end up not meeting them, then you'll be discouraged and likely quit straightaway. Taken in the other direction, if you set too low expectations, then you'll never be motivated enough to start in the first place.

Your expectations may focus on different areas, depending on what you want from a dietary and lifestyle change. Here are some ideas to help jump-start your endeavors to figuring out your expectations:

✔ **Lose fat:** If you want to lose some fat from fasting, determine what amount of fat loss is reasonable. You may choose, for instance, to start with a pound a week. Some experts may even tell you more than a pound a week, but we feel that amount is a little too generous. Through diligent efforts, an overweight person could lose up to 4 to 5 pounds every 30 days, which isn't bad at all.

You can't go into fasting and think that everything is going to change overnight. It takes a while to put on excess body fat, and it takes a while to take it off. There are no quick and easy fixes to losing that fat, but there are proven and reliable processes. Fasting is a proven process. Fasting can get you to your ideal body weight, and it can help you get there more quickly than almost any other dietary and lifestyle change. But you must understand that it's going to take some time.

✔ **Feel healthier:** Feeling healthy is hard to describe, but you'll know it when you feel it. You'll notice a lighter bounce to your step and a more elastic spring in all your joints. The fog in your mind will begin to lift, and your overall concentration will sharpen.

If you have other ailments, such as digestive issues or chronic inflammation, you can expect those to dissipate as well, even within a week.

✔ **Be more energetic:** People who fast report feeling more energetic, more alert, and less irritable. You'll also have more energy to do the activities that you love with friends and family.

Many times people don't know just how bad they feel until they start feeling better. It's hard to notice that you're in poor health when it's been so long since you've ever experienced good health. Let fasting guide you back to good health!

Are these goals realistic for you? Maybe. Maybe not. It depends entirely on the individual and the fasting practice, but in most cases you can reasonably expect to start feeling better on the whole in less than one month.

To establish your own expectations and goals with fasting, consider the following pointers:

✔ **When you start, take baby steps.** We assume that you don't have any prior experience fasting. When you start, go with the flow for the first two to three weeks without setting any expectations at all. Doing so allows you to gather some information and to see how your body responds to fasting.

✔ **After you feel more comfortable fasting, be realistic with long-term goals and expectations.** For example, if in the first two weeks you lose three pounds, then you know that you shouldn't expect to lose more than five pounds a week. If you come out of the first two weeks very disappointed, and likely quit, you never really acknowledge that losing three pounds is still a great success.

Setting realistic goals and expectations is at best a crapshoot without prior data on how your body responds to something. So, hold off for two to three weeks on setting any long-term expectations until you have a general idea of how your body responds.

Thinking long term, not short

When you figure out whether fasting is right for you, you also need to look at the long-term commitment of fasting. Fasting isn't an extreme form of yo-yo dieting. It's a permanent, long-term lifestyle alteration. If you think you're going to look radically different after one fast, you're going to be enormously disappointed.

Fat loss is largely a numbers game. You need only to consistently put out more calories than you take in in order to succeed. Consistently is the most important word. Fasting is one of the best ways to lose fat because it helps you to *consistently* assume a caloric deficit. Fasting helps you lose fat by hacking away at your overall number of calories week by week. It is a slow but sustainable process. Because it's a slow and sustainable process also means that it's a successful process.

Realistically, the shortest amount of time you should expect to see tangible results is three months. Three months is the length of a season, which is a fair amount of time to objectively assess whether or not something is working for you.

Identifying the Fasting Mindset

Success is a habit. And a habit is simply how you go about doing things, over and over. Habits are programmed and are largely unconscious acts (you don't think about them). Because habits are programmed, they're ultimately programmable, which means they can be installed and uninstalled, just like you can install a successful mindset.

In fact, you can classify almost anything as a habit. Happiness, for example, is a habit. And so is misery. Failure too is a habit. And so is success.

The successful fasting mindset (or the habit of success) is positive and optimistic. It's also realistic. In order to change your mindset, you need to monitor and change your thoughts because thoughts beget feelings, feelings beget behaviors, and behaviors beget habits. Having a successful mindset all starts with your thoughts, and these sections give you a mini crash course in psychotherapy to help you avoid negative thoughts and create a positive way of thinking, which can lead to success.

Abolishing a negative mindset

Before you can install your new mindset, you first have to remove your current negative mindset because these negative thoughts lead to habits. A simple way to get rid of your old mindset that isn't working: Stop thinking "I can't" and focus on "I can." You'll act in accordance to your thoughts. If you think you can't, you're right. On the other hand, if you think you can, you're right, so be aware of your thoughts.

To help you eliminate your negative thoughts, use a thought journal. For one week, write down all negative thoughts that you have in a notebook or journal, such as "I look so fat," "I hate the way I look," or "Why did God give me these thunder thighs?" If you're like most Americans, the journal will quickly fill. You're probably not aware of how much negative thinking goes on in your head. Monitoring and recording your negative thinking is the first step toward getting rid of it.

After doing so for a week, begin to identify whenever a negative thought creeps into your mind and replace it immediately with a more positive and compassionate thought. This process requires that you're constantly monitoring your thoughts (which is why the journal is so helpful) so that you can straightaway replace all negative thoughts with positive thoughts. Eventually, and with enough practice, this process will become automatic. So, when you think "I hate the way I look," focus on what you do like about yourself and that you're making a concerted effort to improve the way you look.

Establishing the habit of success

To create a new habit and mindset, you need to start to develop a new way of thinking. To do so, you replace the negative thoughts with positive thoughts. Instead of "I can't" or "I won't," focus on "I can" and "I will." In order for this new way of thinking to stick, you need to do it every day, as much as you possibly can.

If you truly wish to establish the habit of success, you can consciously choose to replace any negative thoughts as quickly as possible with a more positive and compassionate thought. You can consciously change your thoughts until the change becomes an unconscious decision. Then as your thoughts change, your feelings will change. And as your feelings change, your behavior changes. After your behavior changes for the better, you're in a condition to install a healthier, more productive habit.

Consider how you put on your pants. Chances are you put your pants on by putting either your left or your right leg in first. And chances are you do it unconsciously, meaning you don't think about it. To change this habit, you must consciously force yourself to do the opposite, and continue to consciously make this change on a regular ongoing basis until the action becomes unconscious. When it becomes an unconscious decision, you've successfully installed a new habit. Failure is putting your pants on one way. Success is doing it another way. It's a simple change of habit — simple, but not easy.

So instead of saying to yourself, "No way am I ever going to be able to go without food for that long," you can be a bit more compassionate with yourself and say something like "Fasting for that long is no big deal. I've gone that long without food before, and the more I do it, the better I'll get at it." What you'll notice about the positive-thought replacement is that it's both comforting and realistic. You have to say something to yourself that is somewhat believable; otherwise, you won't accept it, and you'll revert to your negative thought.

You can use this technique for all endeavors — business, personal relationships, sports competitions, and so on, although it's particularly useful, if not critical, for optimizing your health. If you want to be healthy, then you need to start acting healthy, even if it feels awkward at first.

Sometimes making the thought change isn't easy. Many psychologists suggest you fake it until you make it, which means in order to program the habit of success, you must forcefully act the way you want to be.

Relying on a buddy with before-and-after photos

Another way to ensure your success is to find what we call an *accountabili-buddy,* someone who is a friend, family member, or coworker who can hold you accountable. When you have an accountabili-buddy, we suggest you exchange before photos and food journals. Sharing your food journal (which should include everything you eat and drink throughout the week) with your buddy at the end of every week will help to keep you motivated and on track.

Whenever we work with clients, one of the first things we have them do is take before photos. We then ask them to stash their before photos away for three months. They aren't allowed to take a single peek at them for ninety days. After the three months, we then take another round of photos and compare them to their before photos. The result is always astonishing, and the clients can hardly ever believe that they looked the way they did three months ago.

We encourage you to do the same thing with your accountabili-buddy. Before you start your fasting journey, take before photos, best done in your bathing suit. Take one shot from the front, one from the side, and one from the rear. Then stash them away somewhere where you can't look at them for three months. After three months of fasting, snap your after photos and compare them to your before photos. You're going to like what you see. We guarantee it.

This technique of before-and-after photos works for a couple of reasons:

- Noticing progress is almost impossible when you see yourself every day. The changes on a day-to-day basis are nearly imperceptible, but you can't miss progress after three months.

- Adhering to your fasting protocol is easier when you have a deadline. Seeing the amount of progress you've made after three months will skyrocket your motivation and increase the likelihood that fasting will become a permanent part of your lifestyle.

Making Fasting Work

You can make this whole business of fasting easier. In addition to developing a positive mindset (which we discuss in the previous section), you don't have to make fasting more difficult than it needs to be. Make sure you select the fasting practice that best suits your schedule and lifestyle. You don't need to push a boulder up a hill, which is what you'll be doing if you choose a fasting practice that doesn't fit your schedule or lifestyle. Let fasting work with you, not against you, by choosing one that best fits your life situation. Check out the chapters in Part II for the fasting program right for you. These sections discuss a few tweaks that can make fasting more practical.

When beginning, you want to fast for an amount of time that will challenge you, but enables you to be successful. For example, although a full 24-hour fast is a great place to end up, it's not exactly the best place to start. If you try to do too much at once, you may feel overwhelmed and likely want to quit altogether. You need to build your confidence and your fasting periods up slowly.

Keeping your mind focused elsewhere

The greatest challenge that comes with fasting is hunger. Over time, you'll figure out how to embrace hunger. And believe it or not, many people who fast discover how to enjoy being in a hungry state. Remember that mindset is everything!

But until you reach that point, you need to keep distracted and to not focus too much on the hunger; otherwise, you'll quickly find yourself reaching for a snack. To some individuals, this tip may sound counterintuitive; to others it's common sense. Our best advice is to keep yourself as busy as possible and to choose to fast on the days where you're most likely to be engaged in some sort of activity that's going to hold your interest.

Some people think that fasting on a busy day can make the entire day more difficult. But others see the hidden advantage, which is distraction. Our experience has shown us that people who fast on their busiest days are the ones who are most successful. When you sit around and have nothing to distract you from your hunger, fasting becomes a more difficult practice than it needs to be.

The activity that keeps you busy doesn't have to be a work-related activity. Games, sports, movement, exercise, and work are all effective for stealing your attention away from hunger. And the more you get into the habit of keeping yourself distracted, the less noticeable the hunger, and the easier fasting becomes. For instance, many of our clients are golfers and have found great success by golfing in a fasted state. For them, golf is an enjoyable and engaging activity so their minds are focused on the game rather than on their stomachs. Furthermore, golf is a low-intensity physical activity, a perfect complement to fasting.

If you want some tricks to help you succeed on your fast, check out www. dummies.com/extras/fastdiets.com.

Committing yourself 100 percent

If you decide to fast, make a commitment to your new lifestyle and then go. To begin the lifestyle change means clearing out your fridge, freezer, and pantry of foods that don't work best within your body. When you take these action steps and restock with the real foods we recommend, you jump-start your body's improvement in every way. Your body begins

- ✔ **Eliminating toxins:** When you eat *nutrient-dense* (foods that have high nutrients relative to their calories), non-inflammatory foods, toxins exit your body through the liver, lungs, intestines, and kidneys.

- ✔ **Losing weight and slaying your sugar cravings:** You're breaking sugar addiction as you eat healthier proteins, carbohydrates, and fats, and your body begins using fat for fuel rather than using sugar and sugary carbohydrates.

- ✔ **Getting your gut health in order:** Every 21 days, your intestinal cells turn over *(regenerate)*. The nutrient-dense, non-inflammatory foods you feed your body during the eating phase of your fast are the best raw materials to form the healthiest cells possible. This regeneration will get you healthy, lean, and strong.

- ✔ **Reducing inflammation:** The healthy fats and clean foods quiet inflammation throughout your entire body. This concept is one of the cornerstones of fasting and eating healthy during your eating window — and throughout your life.

✓ **Rebuilding and healing:** All the structures and functions of your body begin to strengthen when you fast and eat the foods that work best with your body during your eating window.

✓ **Balancing your fatty acids:** Your ratio of omega-6 to omega-3 fatty acids improves greatly when you eat the right fats and oils, which is great for reducing inflammation and healing the body. These healthy fats can give you radiant skin as well.

✓ **Optimizing your metabolism:** The balance of *macronutrients* (which are the protein, carbohydrates, and fat that provide you with energy) helps you create an efficient metabolism.

✓ **Balancing blood sugar:** The foods you're eating during your eating window help stabilize your blood sugar for the long-term.

To do a fast, you don't need special pills or juices. Just make sure all the foods you choose during your eating window are from real sources, with a focus on quality.

Managing your hunger

Keeping your hunger in check is more of an art than a science. It takes some creativity and experimentation, but over time, you can find fun and unique ways to keep hunger at bay. Chapter 14 provides some specific strategies and activities you can do to help you keep your hunger levels low and your energy levels high.

Focusing on the fasting game: Reprogramming with affirmations

When working on understanding and adopting what to eat during your eating window, you need to program yourself for success. Concentrate on not going back to any old foods or habits that may not serve you or past negative experiences you may have had with food. Use your mind to strengthen you, not weaken you. When you develop a strong mind, you'll achieve the ultimate in health and weight loss.

By navigating your mind and emotions toward positive outcomes, you begin to reprogram your mind toward what you want. Look at fasting as liberating rather than overwhelming or difficult, because through fasting and eating the foods we recommend in Chapter 8, you're going to recalibrate your body to look and feel amazing. You'll get leaner and stronger every day.

(continued)

(continued)

A great way to do this is through affirmations, which are healing poems, quotes, verses, and sayings that help you visualize your success.

Write down in a notebook or journal what you want — or who you want to be. We suggest you even take notes or journal with a red pen because the color red subconsciously helps you pick up the message. You can develop your own affirmations or refer to the many books on this topic.

Each morning say your affirmations aloud with intention, before your mind has a chance to fight back. As you read them, move your body to integrate the words into your physiology (so the words become a part of who you are). Say this affirmation as you finish: "I am fasting my way to lean, strong, and healthy."

Soon these affirmations will become ingrained in your cells and part of your identity. Reciting affirmations may seem like a silly or small little habit, but this habit definitely packs some power. Many influencers and leaders that are skilled at getting the outcomes they want use this simple strategy as part of their winning arsenal.

Planning Ahead for Potential Pitfalls and Slip-ups

You're a human being, and mistakes are bound to happen. From time to time, you're bound to give in to temptation. Doing so is okay if it's only from time to time. You can handle mistakes when they happen and mitigate the negative effects of breaking your fast. If you do have a slip-up, remember these important points:

- **Realize that the slip-up isn't the end of the world.** Like any discipline, fasting takes practice, and slip-ups are bound to happen.

- **Keep everything in perspective.** Don't allow one minor slip-up to turn into a cascade down the side of a mountain. If you slip up and break your fast with a snack or a meal, acknowledge it, accept it, and leave it at that. Whatever you do, don't turn it into a 24-hour binge.

- **If you slip up, try to do so with something healthy.** If you absolutely must have something to eat, reach for a source of lean protein (such as salmon, tuna, or chicken) and vegetables (such as spinach, asparagus, or cauliflower) before the bag of potato chips or bowl of ice cream.

We can't stress the importance of this point enough. If you get into the habit of slipping up with poor food choices, then you'll invariably revert to junk food whenever hunger strikes. If you break your fast, you absolutely must get into the habit of doing so with healthy food choices. Done this way, your slip-ups become more of a positive than a negative.

Everything you put into your body matters. Every single piece of food either helps to move you closer toward your goals or farther away. Making the right food choices when you slip up makes all the difference.

✔ **If you do slip up, eat as little as you need to satisfy your urge, and not a smidgeon more.** Don't let a small slip-up be the end of your fast. The key is to satisfy what you absolutely must have with as little as you need, and then continue onward as if the slip-up never occurred. For example, say you're on a 24-hour fast, and at hour 16, you just can't take it anymore and help yourself to a handful of nuts. Just because you ate a handful of nuts doesn't mean you have to forfeit the rest of your fast. Quite the opposite, actually.

The objective is to ensure that you leave the fasted state in a healthy and sensible manner and not to turn something into a calamity that needn't be a one.

All in the family: Kellyann's support system

My parents were a strong foundation for me when it came to healthy eating and exercise. Now in their late 70s, they're an excellent example of the payoff someone can receive when choosing to live a physically active life flecked with an optimistic attitude, mindfulness, and a healthy diet. They're as vibrant as those people in their 40s.

My mother, a beautiful artist, spends her days painting and taking art classes. My father thinks nothing of playing 18 holes of golf without a golf cart! And if that's not inspiring enough, he often carries his own bag, while grinning ear to ear. A few times a week, they *bust it up* in my sister's health center, participating in metabolic/strength training and causing jaw-drops among many of the center's members.

Every day continues to be an exciting adventure for my parents. They *truly* are enjoying life.

Although my sister (she's a doc, too) and I have had somewhat of an impact on our parents' lifestyle choices, my parents have influenced and inspired us as well. And they still do!

My sister and I became doctors, practicing wellness principles. My younger brother obtained a black belt in tae kwon do and has been a jujitsu instructor for more than 20 years. My older brother, a three-time state cycling champion, is an avid cyclist who competes throughout the country. We all have embarked on health-related careers and/or healthy lifestyle practices that were originally set by our parents.

Being a good role model can indeed make a difference for future generations. I look to my two sons to make the most of their lives with healthy lifestyles as well.

Leaving a Fast Early: How to Do So Sensibly

Sometimes life gets in the way. If for some reason you have to stop your fast, we hope you think through the decision before doing so. If you have no other course of action, when you do end a fast, keep these pointers in mind to help so you can get as much from your fast as possible:

- **If possible, end your fast hungry, but not ravenous.** That is, don't try to fast for longer than you're able to at first, because doing so can increase the likelihood of binging post fast. Gradually increase the length of your fasting periods. If you're ravenous when you do end, be careful about binging.

- **Eat high-fiber, low calorie foods.** When coming off your fast, fill up first on food that takes up space with few calories, such as cruciferous vegetables, including broccoli or cauliflower. Doing so can help to initially settle your hunger without consuming too many calories. Stay away from foods with high calories and high fat, such as pizza and burgers.

- **Eat until you're satisfied, not bloated.** You don't have to clean the plate every time. Eat until you're good and satisfied, but put the fork down before you stuff yourself silly.

Part II
Identifying Practical Fasting Practices

Advantages of drinking green tea

Research has shown some well-researched benefits of green tea consumption, which include the following:

- **Antioxidant support:** Antioxidants in green tea (specifically *catechins*) are more effective than even vitamin C and vitamin E at healing oxidative damage in the cells.

- **Metabolism boost:** Green tea provides a gentle but substantial metabolic boost through the stimulation of adrenaline, which results in an increase of *lipolysis* (fat burning) not so different from what you experience while fasting.

- **A decrease in bad cholesterol:** Green tea not only reduces bad cholesterol, but may also help to regulate blood pressure and reduce the risk of hypertension.

- **Good for your teeth:** The antioxidants in green tea help to ward off and even reverse tooth decay.

- **Anti-aging:** The antioxidants and gentle stimulation of green tea work to slow and reverse the biological aging process, which means healthier, more vibrant skin, increased energy, feelings of vigor, and a reduced risk for illness.

Not all teas are created equal. Go with organic when you can and choose only full leaf tea varieties, and not the finely ground-up tea dust.

Head to www.dummies.com/extras/fastdiets for different ways that you can fast.

In this part...

✔ Understand the differences in timing, meals, and philosophies of several of the most popular and widely followed fasting diets, including intermittent fasting, the 5:2 Diet, micro-fasting, and the Warrior Diet.

✔ Discover how long a fast typically lasts — from just over half a day to a full 24-hour period — and tips on how to successfully complete a fast.

✔ Find out which fasting practice fits best with your current lifestyle, obligations, and commitment levels.

✔ See why the commonsense adages of eating breakfast and eating frequently throughout the day can actually hinder your fat-loss and health goals.

✔ Comprehend what you can and can't eat or drink during your fast, as well as the best practices on choosing foods during your nonfasting time periods.

Chapter 4

Dieting Sporadically: Intermittent Fasting

*W*ith intermittent fasting, you're not only taking an occasional break from food, but you're also helping your body find balance in your eating habits, thus freeing yourself from dieting and from compulsive eating behavior. Yes, *intermittent fasting* means abstaining *from* eating from time to time, but it also means freedom *to* eat.

This chapter explains the basic tenets of intermittent fasting, including the upsides and downsides to this type of fasting, when you should fast (and when you shouldn't), how long to fast, what you can and can't eat during the fast, and what you should eat after fasting. Here you can discover how to reap the benefits of intermittent fasting by successfully completing a fast.

Figuring Out What Intermittent Fasting Really Is

Intermittent fasting — or dieting sporadically — simply means you take a break from eating one to two times per week (meaning a full 24- to 32-hour fast), while the rest of the time you follow some basic eating guidelines that you probably already know but unfortunately seldom follow. These guidelines include taking the time to enjoy the foods you eat, eating lots of fresh fruits and vegetables, utilizing herbs and spices instead of salt to flavor food, and eating less overall. The beauty of intermittent fasting is that it's not a diet in the traditional sense. Rather it's a lifestyle change and a sustainable one at that. After you understand how to do it and begin successfully completing fasts, intermittent fasting will get — and keep — you on the right track to a lean and healthy life.

By its very nature, you'll eat less when you abstain from eating one or two times a week with intermittent fasting. Fasting really isn't new to you, although you may not be aware of it. You normally fast on a typical day (most people fast between six and ten hours when they're asleep each night). Just by fasting twice a week and eating as you normally would the rest of the time, you could be cutting your weekly caloric intake by nearly 29 percent, which is a reduction of nearly 600 calories each day of the week. The rest of the time you eat as you normally would, focusing on healthful options, such as the Paleo Diet (see Chapter 8 for more specifics). Even more so, with intermittent fasting, you stop stressing so much about the foods that you do eat.

With so much conflicting health and diet advice all around, the act of eating, which traditionally is one of celebration and community, becomes a stressful occasion. Just take a look at the magazine covers in the checkout line at the grocery store; headline after headline promises the best diets for fast weight loss. One diet espouses the benefits of low-fat foods, another advises cycling your carbohydrate intake. Yet another prescribes severe caloric restriction. Often, these diets' principles conflict with one another, making it impossible to figure out which one is going to work the best. And even more detrimental, they act as quick fixes — diets that you only have to follow for a short amount of time and that aren't sustainable in the long run, setting you up for another weight loss and healthy living failure.

While you take a break from eating with intermittent fasting, you also give yourself a break from scouring through health and fitness magazines and websites trying to find the next new, guaranteed diet plan that gives fast results. And perhaps most importantly, you begin to put a stop to the over-abundance that may well be present in your own life.

Seeing the Pros and Cons to Intermittent Fasting

Intermittent fasting carries a unique set of pros and cons. In these sections, we examine the upsides and downsides, so that you can make an informed decision as to whether or not fasting intermittently is the best approach for you. In brief, we look at why intermittent fasting might be the best fit if you're looking for the most flexible approach to fasting, and why it may not be a good fit if you're new to fasting or not yet ready to tackle a full 24-hour fast.

Intermittent fasting provides many benefits and can help you realize your weight loss goals. However, remember that it's *not* magic. Just because you fast once or twice a week doesn't mean you can gorge on junk food to make up for the calories that you didn't eat while fasting.

Highlighting the pros

Intermittent fasting is a very beneficial practice, is easy to follow, and allows you the flexibility you need for when life happens. By getting to choose and flex your fasting days and selecting when you start your fasting periods, intermittent fasting really can work for you, and you never need to go to bed hungry. It doesn't have any complicated formulas, diet plans, pricey supplements, or special foods that you need to buy.

Intermittent fasting is simple and it's effective. Some of the other benefits to intermittent fasting include the following:

- ✔ **The ability and flexibility to set and change your fasting schedule as time goes on:** You don't need to keep your fast on the same day each week. Really, it doesn't matter when you do it, so long as you do it. You can choose the best time or day to fast. Some people prefer weekends, and others prefer weekdays. Just stop eating for 24 hours, one day a week. The day doesn't matter.

    One full day of fasting is plenty. Fasting for 24 hours allows you to reap the full benefits of fasting. Just don't take the more-is-more approach and fast any longer than 24 hours.

- ✔ **The freedom from continuously planning your day around your next meal:** When you first take a break from eating, you'll likely be astonished by the sheer amount of time that is free in a day. You don't have to plan or prepare meals, at least for one day out of the week. For many people, it's very liberating.

- ✔ **A reduction in weekly food costs:** Not eating for a full day once a week means a lower weekly grocery bill.

> ✔ **An uncomplicated diet plan with no tricky formulas, equations, or costly meal plans:** Intermittent fasting is so easy. You just don't eat for a day. That's it! No counting calories, carbs, or anything of that sort. You don't eat. Period.

We can't stress the benefits of intermittent fasting enough. Scientific studies have also proven time and again its efficacy in terms of weight loss, muscle gain, and insulin sensitivity. Chapter 2 addresses the science behind fasting and how fasting can help improve brain function and immunity to common illnesses, and increase energy levels, muscle growth, and a loss in body fat.

Considering the cons

Unlike some of the other fasting systems (like those in Chapters 5, 6, and 7), the intermittent fasting approach does require at least a full 24-hour fast, which can be difficult, especially if you've never tried fasting before. That's certainly not to say that you won't become accustomed to it. Just be aware that there will be challenges, such as staving off hunger and feeling low energy levels, particularly at first. (Chapters 14 and 15 provide some helpful tips.)

Don't be discouraged by the idea of fasting for 24 straight hours. You can reach many of the benefits of your fast prior to the 24-hour mark. Although you should always strive to complete the full fast when following the intermittent fasting protocol, if on a given day you just feel like you need to end your fast early at, say, 22 hours, that's okay, too.

Grasping the Ins and Outs of Intermittent Fasting

By committing to intermittent fasting, you're committing to abstaining from eating or drinking anything with calories during a set time period one to two times a week. In this style of fasting, your fasts will last at least 24 hours at a time. Although 24 hours may seem like an insurmountable length of time at first, you can make the fast seem less arduous by building up to a full 24-hour fast and by the timing of your fasting periods.

To help you with your intermittent fast, these sections explain what you can do to be effective and what the best time is both to fast and not to fast.

Being successful with your intermittent fast

In order to succeed with your intermittent fast, you first need to be able to embrace those feelings of hunger. Be aware that feeling hungry or wanting to eat aren't true feelings of hunger or deprivation. Your mind is merely telling your stomach to feed because that's what your mind is used to doing. Being able to develop the fortitude to forego food for a short amount of time is incredibly important because only when you stop eating can you go from a fed state to a fasted state and reap all the wonderful benefits of fasting.

If you have never fasted before, being hungry can be very uncomfortable. If you attempt to fast too long on your first couple of tries, you run the risk of breaking the fast by gorging on unhealthy foods, instead of eating healthful and nutritious foods that will help take advantage of the fast that you just completed. (We explain what foods you can eat when breaking an intermittent fast in the "Identifying What You Can and Can't Eat" section later in this chapter.)

When you first start an intermittent fast, you may want to set shorter fast periods, such as fasting for 12 hours, and then increasing the duration each time you complete a fast until you've reached the full recommended 24-hour fast period. Doing so may take several weeks, which is okay. You'll have more confidence in your abilities if you set a shorter fast period and succeed rather than trying to go for the full 24 hours on your first try and failing.

Embarking on a new diet or fitness regimen may feel novel and exciting, but oftentimes that novelty wears off and you find yourself having difficulty sticking to it, and you begin searching for something new. If you find yourself in this situation, make a promise to yourself to stick with fasting for one full month before deciding to try a different approach.

Figuring out the best times to fast

Intermittent fasting is inherently flexible. Because you only need to fast one or two times a week, you can begin your fast at the time that is most convenient for you as long as you ultimately fast for 24 hours.

As a result, you can start your once or twice weekly fast at any time on any day of the week. That means intermittent fasting has no set schedules. You can easily adjust your fasting days for what's best for you. Say, for instance, you're planning on fasting Wednesday evening through Thursday, but a social engagement — dinner with friends — comes up; you simply can start your fast the following day.

When people sleep, they naturally fast. As a result, fasting from dinner to dinner is easiest for most people, meaning if you finish eating at 7 p.m., you can abstain from eating or drinking anything with calories until 7 p.m. the following evening. If you've ever tried going to sleep while hungry, you know doing so can be a challenging feat. But by following a dinner-to-dinner fasting period, you can fall asleep without having to contend with an empty stomach.

Another popular time to begin and end your fast is a lunch-to-lunch fast. If you choose this fasting schedule, you eat lunch, ending at around 1 p.m. and don't eat again until 1 p.m. on the following day.

We do caution against trying a breakfast-to-breakfast fast. This fasting schedule requires you to fall asleep at night on an entirely empty stomach. Although this schedule may work for some people, more than likely you'll be so hungry by the end of the first day that you may break the fast early and with suboptimal food choices, such as with sugary treats or with a desperate, hunger-driven run to the nearest fast-food restaurant.

Intermittent fasting is also flexible over time. When you first begin intermittent fasting, you may find that the lunch-to-lunch fasting period works best for you, but as time goes on and your work and/or personal schedules change, you may find that you need to switch your fast times, which is completely okay. We want you to fast successfully. Flexibility in when you fast is key to making that happen.

Intermittent fasting should work for you, not against you, so experiment with different fasting schedules. You may find a dinner-to-dinner fast too challenging given your work schedule, or that at first, the lunch-to-lunch fast leaves you too hungry at night to fall asleep. Play around with the different schedules and see what works best for you.

Knowing when not to fast

Although intermittent fasting has been proven to burn body fat, ward off illness, improve brain function, and increase your energy (refer to Chapter 2 for more on the benefits of fasting), some times intermittent fasting isn't appropriate. Make sure you use common sense and consult your physician with any questions that you may have about fasting.

If you find yourself in one of the following groups, you shouldn't do intermittent fasting:

- **If you're pregnant or trying to become pregnant:** When you're pregnant or trying to get pregnant, focus on the pregnancy. After pregnancy, if you want to try intermittent fasting, talk with your physician about whether or not fasting is a good option for you.

- **If you're immunosuppressed:** Consult with your doctor first before doing an intermittent fast. Although some very interesting research focuses on the benefits of fasting for people undergoing chemotherapy, you should never begin fasting on your own if you're currently battling cancer, HIV/AIDS, or any other sort of immunosuppressive ailment without first garnering your doctor's approval.

- **If you're diabetic:** Intermittent fasting has shown to positively affect insulin resistance; however, if you're diabetic, fast only under the direct supervision of your healthcare provider.

- **If you're under 18 years old:** Studies on the effects and benefits of intermittent fasting have focused primarily on adults. For this reason, we don't recommend intermittent fasting to children. Intermittent fasting is therefore only appropriate for otherwise healthy adults and adults who have been cleared to fast by their physician.

You should always check with your physician or healthcare provider before starting any diet or fitness plan. He or she can advise you on whether intermittent fasting is a safe option for you.

Identifying What You Can and Can't Eat

Intermittent fasting is the voluntary abstention from any food or drink that contains calories. So during the 24 hours in which you're fasting, you need to be mindful of what you consume and make sure that it doesn't have any unnecessary calories. These sections clarify in plain English what you can and can't eat when you're on an intermittent fast.

Consuming noncaloric drinks

Although you don't eat anything while fasting, make sure that you drink only noncaloric drinks during your intermittent fast, the most important being water. In fact, you should drink a minimum of eight glasses of water, which can help you feel fuller and can ensure you're staying hydrated throughout the day.

Other noncaloric drinks you can consume during your intermittent fast include the following:

- Black coffee
- Black tea
- Green tea
- Herbal teas, such as peppermint, chamomile, or rooibos
- Sparkling water

Keep caffeine to a minimum, if you can because too much isn't good for you or your fast. Our recommendation is not to exceed two cups of coffee in one day (or approximately 200 milligrams of caffeine).

You can easily sneak calories into beverages with milk or sugar, so be careful. Drinking unsweetened tea or not adding half-and-half to your morning cup of coffee can seem difficult at first, but the benefits of intermittent fasting far outweigh the initial discomfort of giving up your routine. If you start to add a dash of cream here or a packet of sugar there, you may soon find that you aren't fasting at all but instead spiking insulin levels and not allowing your body to reap the full benefits of the fasting period. Remember, you're only taking a break from eating once or twice a week so be strong. You can do it.

When first trying out intermittent fasting, some people experience headaches. If you experience headaches, you aren't dehydrated, but rather you're experiencing a common withdrawal symptom. Be mindful of the amount of caffeine you consume during your fast, because caffeine acts as a diuretic. If you consume too many caffeinated beverages while fasting, without drinking enough water or herbal tea as well, you may get a caffeine headache or become dehydrated.

Including supplements

You may also take vitamins or other supplements while fasting. They can include fish oil, a multivitamin, or any other supplement that you normally take on nonfast days.

Some people find that taking supplements, such as a multivitamin, on an empty stomach can make them feel nauseated. If it happens to you, consider only taking vitamins on nonfasting days.

Speak with your physician before taking any supplements or starting any dietary regimen, including intermittent fasting, and be sure to discuss how intermittent fasting may affect any physician-prescribed medications or supplements.

Staying clear of foods with calories

Avoid any food or drink that will cause a spike in insulin because *insulin* is the hormone that regulates whether you store fat or release it. By maintaining low levels of insulin throughout your fast, you ensure that the body has a chance to release — and use — fat stores, rather than continuing to pack fat around the typical trouble areas of your tummy, hips, thighs, butt, and arms. (Chapter 2 discusses insulin in greater depth and how insulin spikes can be detrimental to losing weight.)

Overall, what you can consume and what you can't consume during your intermittent fasting period is pretty simple. If you have to question whether or not you can eat or drink a particular food or beverage while on your fast, chances are you should probably just say "no thanks." After all, you're only passing on that item once or twice a week. What you can't eat or drink during your fast includes the following:

Anything with hidden calories

Be careful of what you put into your mouth during a fast; sometimes calories are hidden in places you don't expect. What we mean is the difference between making and breaking your fast can come down to the cream and sugar you put into your coffee.

Black coffee, black tea, and other approved beverages during your fasting period have minimal calories (2 calories or less) and therefore are allowed. (Refer to the previous section, "Consuming noncaloric drinks," for the list of approved drinks.) Adding sugar or creamer to these beverages constitutes unnecessary calories and therefore isn't allowed during the fast.

Chewing gum, including sugar-free gum

The idea behind chewing gum isn't bad. In fact, evidence suggests that humans have been chewing on the leaves or sap of the gum tree for hundreds of thousands of years. However, you should avoid chewing gum, both regular gum and sugar-free. Regular gum has sugar (and also calories). Regular chewing gum is typically sweetened with corn syrup, which is a form of sugar called glucose. This sugar gives you a rise in blood sugar each time you pop a piece.

Sugar-free chewing gum also makes the list as a fasting no-no because of the artificial sweeteners. Furthermore, a small percentage of the population has a genetic intolerance to phenylalanine, which exists in aspartame, that limits how much phenylalanine they consume. When it comes down to it, you need to ask yourself if the artificially sweetened gum is worth it — or can you get the same benefits by choosing a healthier alternative.

Diet beverages

No matter whether it's diet soda, diet iced tea, or some other kind of diet drink, you want to steer clear of it during your intermittent fast. Although diet drinks (and sugar-free gum) typically don't have more than a few calories, they are restricted to avoid the potentially harmful chemicals that can be found within them and their potentially negative effects on your health. Furthermore, a recent study from Purdue University suggests that diet soda can actually increase insulin levels — another reason to keep clear of the stuff.

Although one of the many great benefits of fasting is weight loss, a goal that noncaloric sweeteners (refer to the nearby sidebar for the specific sweeteners) help many people achieve, fasting is also a time to give your body a break from the chemicals inherent in so many of the drinks (and foods) that you enjoy on a regular basis. On your fast days, take a break from the fake stuff and stick to water, black coffee, unsweetened tea, and other noncaloric and healthful beverages.

Examining the most popular sugar-free sweeteners

Sugar-free sweeteners are found in a wide variety of products, from diet sodas to hygiene products. A 2004 study noted that because of this variety and the unknown amounts of artificial sweeteners that people ingest on a daily basis, the risk of developing cancer from these sugar substitutes shouldn't be underestimated. Therefore, whether or not you're on a fast day, limiting your intake of the following artificial sweeteners is important.

✔ **Aspartame:** Found in many sugar-free foods including diet soda, aspartame gets a particularly bad rap. Studies have shown it can increase appetite, especially the day *after* consumption. (Intermittent fasting works, in part, because of the occasional caloric restriction inherent to this practice. If you overindulge the day following a fast, you may mitigate its efficacy.) In a 2007 study conducted on rodents, aspartame caused cancer in the test subjects. Furthermore, aspartame has also been linked to headaches, migraines, and panic attacks due to its role as an *excitotoxin*, meaning it overstimulates nerve cells in the brain. Some people experience such side effects by consuming products that contain aspartame; others simply don't. But whether or not you're part of the population that dislikes the taste of aspartame and/or experiences any of the negative effects associated with its consumption, enough science proves that aspartame isn't an altogether healthy alternative to sugar.

✔ **Saccharine:** This artificial sweetener has been around since the late 1800s as a calorie-free sugar substitute. Nowadays, its most often recognizable form is in the little pink packets. Saccharine is an organic compound made from petroleum. Studies in the 1970s showed that it caused bladder cancer in rodent test subjects. Due to its potential carcinogenic effects, the USDA moved to ban saccharine entirely, but instead, a compromise was reached and a warning label was added to products containing saccharine, allowing it to stay on the market. The warning label was removed in 2000, but lingering doubts on the safety of this artificial sweetener remain.

✔ **Sucralose:** The FDA approved sucralose (brand name Splenda), which is 600 times sweeter than plain old table sugar, for human consumption in 1998. It's often hailed as a better option for people looking for a noncaloric sweetener, especially because it doesn't seem to have the undesirable aftertaste that many sugar substitutes have.

Sucralose started out as sucrose (sugar), but its chemical makeup was changed, turning it into a substance that the human body can't metabolize. It passes through the body without being used by it and thus having a calorie-free effect on the body. However, long-term studies of sucralose's effects on humans haven't been conducted. As a result, we still advise keeping your sucralose use to a minimum.

✔ **Stevia:** Another sugar substitute that may not have the negative effects of others is

(continued)

(continued)

stevia. *Stevia* is an herb-based, noncaloric sweetener that originated in South America. Liquid stevia can pack a sweet punch; a few drops equal the sweetness in a whole cup of table sugar.

What has made this noncaloric sweetener attractive to consumers is that it's not deemed a part of the artificial crowd in the same way (we just include it here to keep all the sweeteners grouped together).

Rather, stevia is plant-based, has been used globally, and has been deemed safe for diabetics. That said, however, it does have a rather strong underlying taste that may need to be acquired. Is it a taste that *should* be acquired? Well, that's up to you. But as a sugar substitute that must be processed before humans can consume it, we suggest keeping it to small doses.

Coming off the Fast: What Can You Eat?

You've just finished a 24-hour fast. You're hungry. You're ready to eat. And you're proud of yourself for successfully abstaining from any food or drink with calories for the past day. Maybe you want to give yourself a pat on the back for doing so — and you should as long as it's just that — a pat on the back. After you complete a fast, don't congratulate yourself with extra helpings of food or dessert.

You may feel like you deserve a treat for enduring the past 24 hours without food, but get rid of the idea that to treat yourself or celebrate a happy event (or console yourself in the wake of an unhappy one) that you need food.

For many people, food is often the ultimate reward. Get a promotion? Go out for a celebratory dinner. Win the softball league championship? Victory beers and pizza are in order. Get through a particularly bad day at work? Break open the pint of ice cream. After all, you deserve it, right?

But this thinking can have some incredibly negative effects in the long run. Because you can always find reasons to celebrate or reward yourselves, all too commonly you wind up eating a surplus of calories — and typically, high-calorie foods that are unhealthy — on a regular basis.

When you finish your intermittent fast, keep the following pointers in mind when you eat so you don't end up throwing away those 24 hours that you fasted.

Journaling what you eat

The easiest way to keep track of what you eat is to keep a food journal on the days you aren't fasting. Doing so allows you to see exactly what you're eating each and every day. The adage "what gets tracked, gets managed" is true. Try it out for a week: Log everything you eat or drink for seven days. Even on your fast days, you can jot down the noncaloric beverages you drink, as well as what you eat to break your fast.

In your journal, write down what you eat, how much you eat of it (calorie count), and when you eat it. In short, if it goes into your mouth, it goes into your journal with as much detail as possible. The food journal isn't so much a way to make you count calories (although can certainly do that if you have a specific calorie count you want to hit) as it is a way to gently remind you to make better decisions when it comes to food, particularly food quality. By writing down everything you eat, the journal holds you more accountable and will help you make better decisions.

You may not even realize what exactly you put in your mouth each day. A food journal can help you track and manage unhealthy eating habits, from snagging chocolate out of your office mate's candy jar to adding an extra pump of caramel to your daily latte. You may even see that you have a history of this kind of celebratory eating.

Selecting healthful and nutritious food

When you come off a fast, you should eat what you would have eaten if you hadn't fasted. Just make sure you focus on choosing nutritious food, meaning you stay clear of the double bacon cheeseburger with fries and a milkshake. Focus on the effect that each macronutrient (such as carbohydrates, protein, and fat) will have on your post-fast body. If you completed a dinner-to-dinner fast (say, 6 p.m. Wednesday to 6 p.m. Thursday), then you eat dinner. If you fasted lunch to lunch, then you eat lunch. Just make sure that you aren't engaging in any celebratory eating, so pick wholesome foods.

You've spent 24 hours controlling your blood sugar levels. Regardless of what you choose to eat after you begin eating again, your body will experience a change in blood sugar. That's to be expected, but you can mitigate that change by making better food choices. For example, if you end your fast by going out to dinner with friends, you may be tempted to eat the dinner rolls. However, by eating carbohydrates as the very first thing after a fast, you'll experience a rise in blood sugar levels that is different from if you broke your fast with dark leafy greens or protein.

Watch out for what we call weekly food traditions. Maybe you have a friend who partakes in this type of eating or maybe you and your family do. These weekly food traditions involve eating a particular food on a certain day of the week, such as Hoagie Tuesday, Pizza Friday, or Pancakes and Waffles Sunday. Following these traditions can lock you into poor eating habits and make it that much harder to adopt a healthy lifestyle. That's not to say that you should get rid of them entirely, but you should be aware of them and be willing to adjust them in order to meet whatever your weight loss, health, and fitness goals are.

Planning your eating ahead of time

To help mitigate the chances of you eating unhealthy foods when breaking your fast, don't set yourself up for failure. Prepare ahead for what you'll eat and have it readily on hand. Don't wait until the last 30 minutes of your fast to realize you have nothing in the house to eat. Have easy-to-eat but healthful foods available to you at the end of your fast. You may find them especially helpful to have in stock to snack on when you're preparing your first regular post-fast meal.

Some healthy foods that are good to have available post-fast to snack on include

- All-natural jerky (beef, bison, ostrich, and so on)
- Apple slices with all-natural almond butter
- Fresh crudités, such as sliced fresh carrots, celery, cucumber, and broccoli or cauliflower florets (you may pair these with homemade vinegar dipping sauce, if you want; check out the recipes in Chapters 9 and 10 for some dressings)
- Hard-boiled eggs
- Raw unsalted nuts, such as Brazil nuts, cashews, macadamia nuts, and walnuts

Despite their name, peanuts aren't nuts; they're legumes. Although you may not have a full-on peanut allergy, if you experience digestive issues when eating peanuts, as you would with other legumes (such as beans), then limit how much you eat and/or switch to a different food.

To help you plan your post-fast meals in advance, prep the vegetables with which you'll be cooking your next meal. Set aside single servings of raw, unsalted nuts in plastic sandwich bags. Make it as easy as possible to break your fast.

Also, be aware of just how much you're snacking in your post-fast period. Nuts can be especially deceiving because they are so small and easy to eat yet pack a powerful caloric punch. Limit how many nuts you're eating in a given day because of their omega-6 fatty acid content. (Refer to Chapter 8 for more information about omega-6 and omega-3 fatty acids.)

Avoid going grocery shopping toward the end of your fast when you'll probably feel the hungriest. Not only will you probably wind up buying more food than you actually meant to when entering the store, but you'll also more than likely purchase some less-than-choice foods that look especially good through the eyes of an empty stomach.

Head to the grocery store before you begin your fast or on a nonfasting day. Bring a list that includes just the healthful and nutritious items you need (and stick to that list), rather than blindly wandering down the aisles (which is where the packaged and generally unhealthy foods reside). Having a list and sticking to it helps you spend less time and less money in the grocery store. Your wallet and your waistline will thank you. Chapters 9 and 10 provide some recipes that you can prepare for your post-fast meal.

Chapter 5

Taking a Different Approach: The 5:2 Diet

In This Chapter

▶ Understanding what makes the 5:2 Diet a unique fasting method

▶ Figuring out how to stick to 500 or 600 calories on your fasting days

▶ Discovering tips and tricks to make fasting easier and more practical

A relatively new entrant into the world of fasting, the 5:2 Diet aims to do away with the feelings of deprivation and struggle that people so often experience in traditional dieting. Instead, it encourages a modified fasting program in which fasting days are spent, not in completely abstaining from food, but in significantly restricting caloric intake.

The goals of this chapter are to give you a better understanding of the 5:2 Diet and its origins, as well as take a look at what foods you should — and shouldn't — be consuming on and off your fasting days, why the glycemic index is especially important for this type of fasting, and strategies on how to stick to the calorie limits set for your fasting days.

Spelling Out What the 5:2 Diet Is

As we detail throughout this book, fasting methods vary from daily micro-fasts to full 24-hour fasts to the kind of fasting that the 5:2 Diet promotes. Unlike other fasting methods, the 5:2 Diet isn't fasting in the traditional sense. We refer to it as a modified fasting program because, in this method, you break up your fasts between meals, meaning you still eat two — although quite small — meals during your biweekly fast days and won't be completely abstaining from food.

Some of the fasting methods we describe in other chapters in Part II require abstaining from all food during your fasting periods; however, in the 5:2 Diet, you still get to eat on your fasting days. You'll simply restrict your daily caloric intake to either 500 calories (for women) or 600 calories (for men).

In essence, the 5:2 Diet actually promotes extreme caloric restrictions twice a week, not strict abstention of eating food and calorie-laden drinks. And the other five days of the week, you go about your usual eating routine. These sections take a closer look at the 5:2 Diet and examine the glycemic index, which is an important concept to better understand how the 5:2 Diet works.

Uncovering this diet's characteristics

One of the perks of the 5:2 Diet is that you aren't dieting most of the time, and the research has shown that this type of fasting style is as effective in weight loss as long-term calorie restriction. Unlike fasting on occasion, daily calorie restriction over the long term typically leaves its followers feeling deprived. As a result, they commonly fall off the wagon and don't get back on again until they come across another fad diet that promises quick fat loss. With the 5:2 Diet, you eat as you normally eat five days a week. Twice a week, you greatly restrict your calories to just 500 (for women) or 600 calories (for men).

For example, say you ate your last meal at 8 p.m. on Sunday. The following morning you eat a small breakfast (really nothing more than a healthy snack; refer to the later section, "Figuring Out What You Can Eat" for what is appropriate to eat during your fast day meals), and then you have another small meal sometime that evening. When you wake up Tuesday morning, it's back to business as usual. You return to your regular eating patterns, not to fast again until your second fast day that week.

For the calories that you do eat while on your modified fasting days, choose ones that won't raise your blood sugar too much. The reason for this is twofold:

- ✔ Fasting can give your body a rest from having to pump out insulin and thus raising your blood sugar levels.
- ✔ Any food you eat will have an effect on your blood sugar, so if you spike it too much too quickly, you'll experience the dreaded blood sugar crash and may not be able to complete a successful fast.

Because of variations in body weight, hormones, and other factors, women and men have different caloric limits on the 5:2 Diet fast days. Women are limited to 500 calories, whereas men are limited to 600 calories. We help you get started with these meals. Chapters 9 and 10 provide more than 55 recipes that you can try.

We also include a few free recipes online at `www.dummies.com/extras/fastdiets` for you to add to your cooking repertoire for your fasting days.

The 5:2 Diet, like other fasting methods, can help do the following:

- ✔ **Activation of the body's repair genes:** When fasting, a process in the body, called *autophagy,* gets switched on. Autophagy means to self eat, so in this repair process the body begins to break down and dispose of old, tired cells, making way for new, healthy ones.

- ✔ **Better moods:** The 5:2 Diet can increase the production of a protein called brain-derived neurotrophic factor (BDNF). Studies have shown that increased levels of BDNF can positively affect the brain, and therefore mood, in much the way that sustained antidepressant medication can.

- ✔ **Increased insulin sensitivity:** The 5:2 Diet helps the body use insulin more effectively, meaning that you don't need to produce as much insulin to get the same amount of work done. By using insulin more effectively, you place less stress on your pancreas, as well as head off the negative effects that too much insulin can cause, such as accelerating the aging process.

- ✔ **Reduction of insulin-like growth factor (IGF-1) levels:** IGF-1 is a hormone that humans produce. The variances in levels present in children help determine growth and future height. However, over time, it's beneficial for adults to have lower levels of IGF-1 because higher levels later in life are correlated with an increased risk of cancer, as well as premature aging.

  Fasting periodically seems to decrease IGF-1 levels in adults, potentially reducing the likelihood of developing common diseases that are associated with age, such as diabetes and cancer. Thus, although it doesn't guarantee immortality, fasting on occasion may give you a taste of the Fountain of Youth.

- ✔ **Weight loss:** The 5:2 Diet includes a decrease in body fat percentage and an increase in lean muscle mass.

Grasping the importance of the glycemic index on the 5:2 Diet

Understanding the blood sugar's effect on the body and the glycemic index of various foods will go a long way in ensuring the successful completion of a fast. The *glycemic index* (GI) is an indicator of how quickly your body's blood sugar will rise after eating a particular food. Because carbohydrates affect blood sugar to a much greater effect than proteins or fats, the GI deals mostly with foods that are higher in carbs but don't have a sizable protein or fat content (of course, there are exceptions to this rule). Blood sugar levels matter because the higher your blood sugar is, the more insulin your body produces. And when your insulin is turned on, your body simply can't — and won't — burn fat. So instead, it stores it, increasing your risk for weight gain, diabetes, metabolic syndrome, and even cancer.

The GI attributes a number that is affected not only by what types of carbohydrates you eat, but also by how much you eat. This is called the *glycemic load* (GL). You can derive the GL with this equation:

$$\text{Glycemic Load (GL)} = \frac{\text{GI} \times \text{carbohydrates (in grams)}}{100}$$

In the GI, each food gets a score out of 100. Stick to food choices that have a score of less than 50 or a GL score less than 20 because foods with a low GI/GL don't cause such a rapid surge in blood sugar. They're slower to digest and absorb in the body, thus helping to avoid a flood of insulin entering the bloodstream.

Furthermore, when talking about GI/GL, not all carbohydrates are created equal. It probably doesn't come as a surprise to anyone that a pear has a considerably lower GI than, say, pancakes slathered in maple syrup. Some foods have GI and GL scores that you might not expect. For example, take dark chocolate. Fifty grams, or 1.8 ounces, of the bittersweet stuff has one of the lowest GI scores — a mere 23. On the other hand, one ounce of breakfast rice cereal has a GI score of 89.

The GI is important when you're fasting on the 5:2 Diet because the fact that higher GI/GL–scoring foods will encourage your body to release insulin and store fat; the inevitable blood sugar crash that comes after eating a high glycemic food will only make fasting that much more difficult. You'll wind up with that uncomfortable empty feeling in your stomach and want to eat again, rather than enjoying longer levels of feeling full and satisfied if you choose foods that are lower on the GI/GL scale.

Fasting paired well with the Paleo Diet can help improve your results. You can't go wrong trying to stick to Paleo-friendly foods while on both your fast and nonfast days.

Only foods that have sizable carbohydrate levels are measured with the GI. That means that foods such as most nuts, eggs, and other protein- and fat-rich foods don't have a GI or GL score, which also means that they won't wreak havoc on your blood sugar levels.

Table 5-1 lists some Paleo-friendly foods with low GI/GL scores that are good for your two fasting days each week on the 5:2 Diet. On your nonfasting days, you can still reach for these foods as a snack to keep your GI/GL levels low.

Table 5-1	Fasting Day Food Choices with Low GI/GL Scores		
Food	*GI*	*GL*	*Portion Size (grams)*
Apple	34	5	120
Banana	47	14	120
Carrots	35	2	80
Cashews	25	5	50
Grapefruit	25	3	120
Orange	31	3	120
Prunes	29	10	60

 When planning out your fasting day foods, be sure to check serving sizes. Because you're only allowed 500 calories (for women) or 600 calories (for men) while following this diet, it can be all too easy to go over your allotted calories, if you don't keep serving sizes in check. You can also search online for food calculators that can help you figure sizes of different foods.

Naming the Upsides and Downsides to the 5:2 Diet

The benefits of the 5:2 Diet are similar to other fasting methods, but some people may not find it as restrictive as, say, the full 24-hour, no-calorie intermittent fasting method that we discuss in Chapter 4. These sections examine the upside and downside to the 5:2 Diet.

The pros of the 5:2 Diet

The 5:2 Diet aims at promoting a healthy and, most importantly, sustainable lifestyle. In this fasting method, you need only to fast twice per week, but unlike other fasting methods, due to its modifications, you'll most likely never go more than 12 hours without eating — and much of your fasting time will occur during sleeping hours.

Some of the pros of the 5:2 Diet include the following:

✔ **You'll never go a full day without eating.** With the start of a new week, having your first fast day fall on Monday may make the most sense for you. But again, pick what works best for you. Just know that you never have to fast for a full day.

✔ **You have flexibility in choosing which days to fast each week.** Those days may vary from week to week, depending on your engagements and obligations. You may find that fasting not from dinner to dinner but from lunch to lunch is most convenient for you. You're allowed to do so. While following the 5:2 Diet, you're encouraged to make it your own. Play with what days and times work best for you. It's more important to complete two successful modified fasts per week than to force yourself into following a rigid schedule of fasting days/times. To that end, because family and social functions typically occur on Saturdays and Sundays, you may find it best to avoid fasting on the weekends.

To avoid getting burnt out on fasting, try not to fast on consecutive days. The emotional and psychological challenges that a back-to-back fast pose may set you up for failure or for an overly indulgent feast on your next day back to normal eating. Besides, as the science has shown, the majority of fasting benefits are had within the first 16 hours. There's no need to push further and make yourself miserable.

✔ **You have the freedom to enjoy food without guilt with common sense.** Because the 5:2 Diet only requires a biweekly fast, you're left with five days in which to eat as you normally would eat. However, we caution that doing so doesn't mean overcompensating or treating yourself for having made it through your fast days. This fasting method works on the premise that you're greatly restricting your weekly caloric intake.

Though you may feel like you've earned it, don't go hog wild on your nonfasting days. Eat sensibly, and don't try to make up for the calories you didn't eat by piling on second — or third — helpings, treating yourself to extra dessert, or by grazing constantly throughout the day. If you try to make up for those calories in the other five days, you won't be getting the benefits of the 5:2 Diet. Let fasting work its magic!

✔ **You experience a reduction in body fat.** Because your weekly calorie consumption will be lower, you can expect an overall reduction in your body fat levels in a safe and reasonable manner.

✔ **It's uncomplicated with no tricky rules to follow.** You simply eat as you normally would five days out of the week. The other two days, you stick to either 500 calories (for women) or 600 calories (for men).

As with all fasting methods, expect opposition. If it's one of your biweekly fasts, expect doughnuts to show up at the office or your friend to invite you out to an impromptu happy hour. Life happens, but remember, whatever you're craving or confronted with on a fast day will be there tomorrow. Delayed gratification is enhanced gratification.

And the cons

On the 5:2 Diet you don't abstain from food entirely; you simply restrict how many calories you eat some of the time. You still get to eat breakfast and dinner on your fasting days, although the meals are quite small. Here are a couple disadvantages of the 5:2 Diet:

- ✔ **You don't achieve a full fast.** On the 5:2 Diet you don't completely abstain from food on your fasting days, which means that you still experience a rise in blood sugar during your fast. A rise in blood sugar can stall fat loss. It can also make you uncomfortably hungry in the middle of your fast as your body comes down from the rise in blood sugar it experienced after having a small meal.

- ✔ **You may experience an arousal in hunger.** Some people have reported that eating 500 or 600 calories on a fast day makes them hungrier. Over time, as you dedicate yourself to full fasting, rather than a restricted fasting program such as the 5:2 Diet, you may find that you adjust to fasting and that your feelings of hunger subside. However, the 5:2 Diet may prolong that adjustment period.

Figuring Out What You Can Eat

Although the 5:2 Diet allows you to eat during your fast days, what you eat matters, specifically in terms of choosing foods that have low GI scores and are able to keep you feeling sustained.

Overall, a general rule that you can use when figuring out what you can eat on your fast days is to pick those foods that are highest in nutritional value and that will keep you feeling satisfied for the longest period of time. Focus on foods high in protein and choose your carbohydrate sources wisely. Opt for carbs that are complex and thus slow burning, rather than simple and quick-burning, such as breads, pastries, and other junk food.

Choosing foods that spike your blood sugar unnecessarily will make completing your fast that much more difficult. If you've ever experienced a sugar crash, then you know just how unpleasant it can be. Usually, to compensate for such a surge — and then decline — in blood sugar, people either feel like they need to take a nap or that they need to eat something more wholesome and sustaining, like a protein-rich, low-carb meal.

If you happen to find yourself in this situation on a fast day, you run the risk of using up your daily caloric limits on less-than-optimal food choices and then, when the inevitable seems to happen and you're uncomfortably hungry and maybe even a little light-headed, you may wind up going over your 500- or 600-calorie limits just to try and make yourself feel better. Before you know it, you've just negated the fast entirely.

Chapters 9 and 10 provide plenty of recipes for the 5:2 Diet to help you make smarter fast-day food choices and to keep you motivated and on track. In the following sections, you can discover how to stick to your 500- or 600-calorie limits on your fasting days, as well as some tips you can employ to make sure you have a successful fast.

Sticking to 500 or 600 calories

The 5:2 Diet allows 500 calories to women and 600 calories to men for the two modified fasting days each week. But what does 500 or 600 calories look like? Well, depending on your food choices, they may not look like much. That's where your understanding of the GI, as well as knowing how to make optimal food choices, is the key to your 5:2 Diet success.

On your fasting days, you should choose foods that keep you satisfied and that also stay within the 500- or 600-calorie per day limits. You can do this by selecting foods that are higher in protein and that have low GI scores. This strategy can help keep your blood sugar on an even keel and keep you feeling satiated.

Choosing foods that have a low GI score and/or that are higher in protein will make sure that you don't experience any wild blood sugar swings, subsequent food cravings, or that uncomfortable empty feeling in your stomach.

Doing so doesn't mean that you have to live on a high protein, low carbohydrate diet forever, but on your two fasting days each week, we do advocate choosing those types of foods.

Furthermore, remember that eating 500 or 600 calories on your fasting days doesn't guarantee that you won't be hungry at all. When you consider how much you eat during the day or what kinds of foods you typically eat, 500 or 600 calories is really just a drop in the bucket. For example, if your typical morning involves a large sugar-laden latte and a bagel with cream cheese from your favorite coffee shop, you may be consuming your entire fasting day's caloric limits before you're even halfway done with breakfast. Not only that, due to the high GI scores coupled with the moderate to low amounts of protein in those foods, the rise (and fall) in blood sugar that you'll inevitably experience will make it that much more difficult to complete a successful fast.

On the other hand, instead of buying your typical high carbohydrate to moderate-to-low protein breakfast, you choose a cup of black coffee or green tea, a hard-boiled egg, one strip of bacon, and a bowl of strawberries, you'll have consumed less than 250 calories, which isn't even half of your fasting day caloric limit. Even better, you've now chosen an all-around healthier breakfast, you'll stay fuller longer, *and* even when you start feeling hungry again, it will be a mild, tolerable feeling, not a crash-and-burn one.

Here are plenty of other tips you can employ to ensure your successful completion of two fasting days per week:

- **Fasting days are not no-fat days, but they are low fat.** So apply healthy fats judiciously (for example, a teaspoon of olive oil on a mixed-green salad rather than an unmeasured amount that drenches everything).

- **If you need that full-stomach feeling, opt for salad.** Overdoing your caloric limit on dark leafy greens is difficult, so you can eat extra spring mix or baby spinach leaves. Just be sure to check how much healthy fat you're adding.

- **Opt for healthy fats.** Whether you're on a fasting day or not, be sure to opt for healthy fats, such as extra-virgin olive oil, coconut oil, walnut oil, avocado oil, ghee, or organic butter from grass-fed cows. Check out Chapter 8 for more information.

- **More flavor equals more satisfaction.** The more flavorful a food is, the more satisfied you'll feel eating it. Adding some lemon or orange juice or some citrus zest to your meals can add that flavorful punch to really brighten the foods you're eating and make them more enjoyable.

- **To get the most accurate calorie count, weigh and measure your food after it's been prepared.** Doing so does require a kitchen scale. Kitchen scales are relatively inexpensive. You can purchase one online or in most stores that have a cooking/kitchen section.

- **Avoid white starchy carbohydrates on fasting days.** These white carbs, which include white bread, white rice, pasta, and white potatoes, have high GI scores. If you eat them, you'll experience a not-so-welcome insulin surge and blood sugar crash. Instead, stick to fresh fruits and vegetables to help curb your carb cravings.

- **Drink plenty of fluids.** Thirst can often mask itself as hunger. So grab a cup of herbal, green, or unsweetened black tea, a cup of black coffee, or a big glass of water and see how you feel afterward. Doing so not only can help fill your stomach, but it can also take your mind off the hunger. The human body is more than 70 percent liquid, so drink at least eight cups of fluids — especially water — each day. On fasting days, we recommend drinking even more fluid than that, in the range of 10 to 12 eight-ounce glasses.

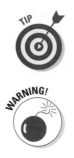

Want something refreshing to drink that isn't plain water, coffee, or tea? Try infusing filtered water with cucumber and mint or strawberries. Add some ice (but if you're in the middle of a fast, skip eating the fruit) and enjoy!

Steer clear of alcoholic beverages on your fasting days. A 2012 study found that many Americans consume more than 300 calories per day from alcohol. That's a lot of empty calories when you're limited to 500 or 600 on your two weekly fasting days.

Eating on nonfasting days

Fasting should be a part of an overall healthy lifestyle, so when it comes to your nonfasting days, don't think of them as a free-for-all. At the same time, because you're fasting, you don't need to feel restricted in your diet either. The key is *not* to try to make up for the caloric deficit you experienced on your fasting days. So don't go hog wild and consume extra helpings of dinner or decide to splurge on a double scoop of ice cream.

The truth is, as hungry as you may feel when you first start out fasting (whether you commit to the 5:2 Diet or another fasting method mentioned in the chapters in Part II), as you and your body become acclimated to fasting, you probably won't feel like overindulging on your nonfasting days. Studies have shown that participants who fasted actually didn't overeat on their non-fasting days, which underscores the important fact that fasting will help you control your appetite, not push it into the extreme.

So instead of obsessively eating (or not eating) certain foods, you'll be able to free yourself from feelings of guilt and deprivation and will be able, instead, to simply enjoy the foods you do eat. Effectively, by freeing yourself from these negative feelings, you'll put an end to what is known as the *disinhibition effect* — that is, the effect that occurs when you overly restrict the foods you eat, which makes you want them all the more. For example: You forbid yourself from eating pasta and wind up gorging on it because of the restriction you placed on yourself not to eat it.

If you aren't restricting the foods you eat on your nonfasting days, you can focus on eating the Paleo Diet for all-around health and vitality. So on your nonfasting days, as well as your fasting ones, we advocate doing away with refined grains, processed sugar, legumes, and most dairy. Chapter 8 provides ideas and tips on how to get your kitchen ready for the fasting lifestyle.

You can utilize the GI even on your nonfasting days. Although you shouldn't feel like you must overly restrict yourself outside of your biweekly fasts, opting for low glycemic, healthful foods throughout the week can get you to your health and weight-loss goals that much faster. The simple goal is to go back to eating as you normally would when you aren't fasting. Don't overindulge and don't gorge. Simply eat as you would to maintain your current body weight, and let fasting works its magic on your metabolism and your body composition. Listen to your body and know when to say when.

Identifying the No-No Foods

With a 500- to 600-calorie limit on your fasting days, you really do have to be judicious in what foods you're consuming. That's why the GI becomes especially important, as we note in the earlier section, "Grasping the importance of the glycemic index on the 5:2 Diet." Stick to foods and beverages that are high in protein and have low GI scores. You'll feel fuller longer and won't experience that dreaded sugar crash and empty-stomach feeling.

Some foods and beverages to stay away from on your fasting days include the following:

- **Typical high-carbohydrate foods, such as pizza, pasta, white rice, and bread:** Not only are high-carbohydrate foods full of empty calories, but they also have high GI scores, meaning they wreak havoc on blood sugar levels. Sudden fluctuations in blood sugar levels will make fasting much more difficult and will negate fasting benefits, such as fat loss and increased insulin sensitivity.

- **Anything with refined or processed sugars in it (table sugar, high fructose corn syrup, agave nectar, and so on):** As you are trying to avoid filling your caloric limits on your fasting days with empty calories, don't waste those 500 or 600 calories on simple sugars. Even honey and maple syrup — two sweeteners that are better choices overall when it comes to satisfying your sweet tooth (but always in moderation) — should be nixed for the two days a week that you're fasting. If staying away from the sweet stuff is tough, just remember: It's only a couple times a week that you have to say no thanks. Another added bonus to this is that giving up sugar a couple times a week will help you finally slay the sugar demon and break free of this highly addictive substance. (See the nearby sidebar about agave nectar for more information.)

Be careful about adding sweeteners and such to your coffee. Although a cup of black coffee has a negligible five calories, a 16-ounce mocha has more than 260 calories — 330 calories if you add whipped cream.

✔ **Soda (regular or diet), sports drinks, or juices:** Americans typically get 140 to 180 calories per day from sugary drinks, like soda and sports drinks. Avoid drinking the diet versions as well.

✔ **Alcohol:** A 2012 study found that, on average, Americans consume 300 calories per day in alcoholic beverages. It may not seem like a lot, but consider how much it can add up to in a week. Besides, many people are consuming much more than that each day. A 5-ounce glass of red wine has 125 calories. A regular 12-ounce beer contains more than 150 calories, and a double vodka and diet cola packs a whopping 258 calories. So imbibing in just one of these drinks can take a serious chunk out of the caloric limits on your fasting days.

✔ **Junk food, including chips, candy, pretzels, fruit snacks, buttery popcorn, and so on:** One of the many benefits of fasting is the cleansing effect it has on the body. Consuming junk food, which is notoriously full of nutritionally subpar ingredients, on your fasting days will only put the toxins that you're trying to rid your body of back inside. Instead, stick to whole, natural, and preferably unpackaged foods during your fast days.

Staying away from agave nectar

You should avoid consuming agave nectar as a sugar during your fasting periods. Agave nectar has enjoyed a boost in popularity over the past few years because it has been deemed a decent sweetening choice for diabetics because it has a lower Glycemic Index/Glycemic Load score than other sweeteners. However, agave nectar isn't all that healthy.

Agave nectar, or agave syrup, is made from the root of the agave plant (the same plant that tequila is made from). It's heavily processed, man-made, and very high in fructose. In fact,

nowhere in nature does such a high fructose-to-glucose sugar ratio occur. So although high fructose corn syrup contains 50 percent fructose and table or cane sugar has 50 percent fructose, agave nectar can contain up to a whopping 92 percent fructose.

The human body isn't designed to handle such large amounts of fructose very well. In response to so much fructose, the body may convert it to triglycerides or inhibit your ability to absorb other nutrients.

Knowing When to Fast and Not to Fast

Before you start the 5:2 Diet or any other fast, make sure you talk to your physician or health professional about fasting, its benefits and drawbacks, and the status of your health. If after doing so, you decide to follow the 5:2 Diet, the following explains when to fast. We also discuss here who should avoid the 5:2 Diet.

Figuring out what days and times to fast

The 5:2 Diet prescribes two days of modified fasting and five days free from calorie counting. When deciding which days during the week to fast, understand that you may have to be flexible. What worked for you last week may not, due to social engagements or other obligations, work for you this week. The key is to choose two nonconsecutive days in which to fast. So for example, if you fasted on Monday, don't fast again until Wednesday or later in the week, giving you at least one full day between fasting periods.

By choosing nonconsecutive days, you won't feel emotionally deprived of food and thus have a better chance of sticking with the program long-term. The 5:2 Diet is aimed at doing away with the feelings of deprivation, anxiety, and guilt that come with so many mainstream diets. *Remember:* Fasting, no matter the method that you choose, isn't a traditional diet; it's a lifelong behavioral change, and the longer you do it, the easier and more fulfilling it will become.

If you decide to fast on a Monday and a Thursday one week, you now just have to decide how long you'll fast for. You'll optimally fast for 16 hours at a time, which has been found to be the sweet spot in fasting — you get the full benefits of a longer fast without the difficulties of completing a longer fast (compared to a fast that goes on for 24 hours or more). But doing so may be challenging with the 5:2 Diet because you break up your caloric limits between breakfast and an evening meal.

However, you may find it easier on your fasting days to get all your calories in one meal. It's really up to you. The 5:2 Diet allows for as much flexibility as all the other fasting methods that we describe in this book. The key is to play around with the fasting method of your choosing, but remember, stick to one particular method for three months before you try another one. Three months is the sweet spot when it comes to giving your body a chance to respond to the fasting method of your choosing and really seeing results from it.

Identifying who shouldn't do the 5:2 Diet

Some people shouldn't fast on the 5:2 Diet, including the following:

- ✔ **Pregnant women:** More research must be done to determine whether or not fasting is safe for pregnant women, and until scientists prove that fasting is healthy during this time of your life, don't fast.

- ✔ **Children:** Because children are still developing physically and mentally, they don't need any nutritional stresses. Although the occasional fast helps decrease the levels of IGF-1 in adults (which helps to promote overall health and longevity), during the formative childhood years, humans naturally have higher levels of IGF-1 to help them grow and develop properly. Never encourage fasting in anyone under the age of 18.

- ✔ **People with medical conditions:** If you have any underlying medical conditions, such as HIV/AIDS, cancer, diabetes, or an eating disorder, fasting probably isn't a wise choice.

If you're a reasonably healthy adult looking to lose some body fat, feel revitalized, and live an all-around healthier lifestyle, then the 5:2 Diet may very well be a viable option for you.

Chapter 6

Micro-Fasting: The No-Breakfast Solution

Micro-fasting is another type of fasting lifestyle that you may want to embrace. Despite its growing popularity, the practice is nothing new. In fact, in 1911 Upton Sinclair wrote a book entitled *The Fasting Cure*, in which he advocated this very approach.

Micro-fasting is mostly for people who want to dabble in fasting more frequently, but not so intensively at any one time. Hence, micro-fasting serves as a general introduction to the world of intermittent fasting (which we discuss extensively in Chapter 4). Micro-fasting isn't too demanding, so to speak.

Micro-fasting, like the Warrior Diet that we discuss in Chapter 7, restricts the amount of time that you're allowed to eat in a day. What makes micro-fasting unique is that it's shorter lived than regular fasting with more frequent bouts of fasting, usually lasting anywhere from 12 to 20 hours, and practiced multiple times a week, if not every day. For example, the most common approach to micro-fasting restricts your eating to an eight-hour window, which leaves you with a 16-hour fasting period. In other words, it's 8 hours on and 16 hours off.

Micro-fasting is very good for you, because it produces all the same tremendous health benefits to be had from intermittent fasting, but it does so in a more lenient manner because the fasting periods aren't so extensive.

This chapter helps make that introduction a bit easier by discussing the ins and the outs of micro-fasting to help you decide if this approach is a good fit for you. Although several different variations of fasting exist, including micro-fasting, no one fasting practice is better than another. The best fasting practice is the one that works for you and your lifestyle. Peruse the other chapters in Part II for other fasting program options.

Tackling the Pros and Cons

Just like all the other fasting practices available to you, micro-fasting also has its pros and cons. The good news: Most people find micro-fasting the most user-friendly of all the fasting practices, even more so than the 5:2 Diet that we discuss in Chapter 5.

Here are the most prominent pros of micro-fasting:

- **Shorter fasting periods may make it easier.** For people who simply aren't ready to tackle a full 24-hour fast (as in intermittent fasting, see Chapter 4), or perhaps just don't want to, micro-fasting has greater appeal, because the fasting period lasts only up to 16 hours. This shorter fasting period makes the whole business of fasting much easier, or at the very least, much more accessible to the newcomer.

- **More frequent bouts may be more effective.** Another advantage of micro-fasting is that you perform the activity more frequently than you would if you were following the full 24-hour fasting protocol. Fasting isn't always a more-is-better activity. If that were true, then why not fast indefinitely? Oh yeah, because you would die. Obviously, you need a delicate balance between eating and not eating for optimum health. But fasting more frequently, not necessarily for longer periods, may very well be enormously beneficial. With micro-fasting, you can practice it every day of the week if you want. You can reasonably deduce that the more often you micro-fast, the more often you reap the benefits of micro-fasting, which perhaps makes micro-fasting a more effective approach. Although scientists haven't conducted any comparative studies on the various modalities of fasting, we're willing to bet that the benefits are greater for more frequent fasting, up to a point.

- **You can time your workouts.** Micro-fasting lends itself uniquely to fasted exercise. In other words, you can time your workouts at the end of your micro-fasting period to boost the positive effects from exercise. When timed right, micro-fasting can greatly enhance the effects of your exercise, which is more difficult to do with some of the other methods in this book. Check out the "Timing Your Exercise with Micro-Fasting" section later in this chapter for additional information.

- **It's more flexible.** You can perform micro-fasting every day, but you don't have to perform it every day, which means it lends itself well to people who seek flexibility, because you may pick and choose the days that you practice micro-fasting. You can start out micro-fasting two to three days to produce tremendous results. Even better, you can spread out these days a week throughout the week depending on what works best for you, which means you can micro-fast a few days in a row, every other day, or in clusters, whatever fits into your schedule.

✔ **You can enjoy social meals.** With micro-fasting, you really only give up breakfast, which means you don't have to forfeit what many people commonly refer to as the most social meal of the day — dinner. Some people have trouble with intermittent fasting because they feel they're unable to socialize if they're not eating. Although we don't think the whole not being able to socialize thing is necessarily true, we recognize that it's a problem for some people, and for them, micro-fasting may very well be the best solution.

And here are a few of the cons to micro-fasting:

✔ **Shorter fasting periods may be less effective.** Studies have shown that the majority of benefits to be had from intermittent fasting occur within the first 12 to 16 hours of a fast. So although micro-fasting is shorter lived than some of the other fasting practices that we mention in this book, you can still reap the same rewards. You just won't reap as many of those benefits at any one time. Evidence suggests that a person can receive marginal benefits when prolonging a fast from 24 to 32 hours. These benefits are simply more of what you're already getting, such as increased lipolysis (fat burning) and natural growth hormone.

✔ **More frequent bouts may make micro-fasting more difficult.** Fasting more frequently, even for shorter periods of time, may be more challenging to some people than fasting just once or twice a week for a full 24 hours. It ultimately depends on the individual and his or her particular preferences. When working with our clients and patients, we have found the majority seem to prefer the convenience of micro-fasting, but some clients still find it easier to opt instead to fast for 24 hours once or twice a week.

✔ **You don't eat breakfast.** The most important aspect to micro-fasting, and perhaps the most controversial, is the regular omission of breakfast, because your eating window occurs later in the day so that you can ride the fasting wave while you sleep. When micro-fasting, you can expect to fast through the morning hours and maybe a little bit of the early afternoon.

Breakfast often plays an important social function, especially in families who like to start the day with some time together around the table. However, just because you're micro-fasting and can't eat food during the morning hours doesn't mean you're ineligible to participate in the social activities of breakfast. You still can sit at the breakfast table with your family or roommates and converse in the mornings. If you absolutely must have something in front of you, then nurse a cup of hot tea or coffee. To understand why breakfast isn't necessary, refer to the next section.

Because the masses unfortunately are highly uneducated with fasting, they — including your family, friends, and peers — may not understand why you're not eating all day. This constant questioning and nagging can get annoying. In fact, this social misunderstanding has turned many people away from the practice of fasting, which is highly unfortunate but a reality. Micro-fasting makes fasting easier, because you don't go for a full 24 hours without food, so you only have to put up with people asking why you're skipping breakfast, but not lunch or dinner. This social obstacle is small, but oftentimes significant. For years we have hoped that most people would gain knowledge of all the marvelous benefits to be had from fasting. But now we know that most people can't absorb knowledge any more than water can absorb oil.

Discovering the Truth about Breakfast

Every night while you sleep you enter into a fast, but as soon as you wake up and eat breakfast, you turn off that fast, and, in turn, miss out on all the wonderful benefits to be had from fasting through the morning hours. The idea that breakfast is a necessity, or the most important meal of the day, is propaganda populated and perpetuated by food companies, specifically cereal companies. Eating breakfast is no more a necessity to life than is getting your toenails painted. That's to say breakfast is a luxury, one that everyone can live without and one that everyone would actually be better off doing without it.

Making breakfast a necessary start to your day actually doesn't make sense for a couple reasons:

- **Most breakfast foods aren't nutritious.** In fact, most breakfast foods suck. They're downright terrible for you. Pancakes, waffles, and cereals are some of the most sugar-laden and nutritionally devoid calories that you can stuff into your body. It's a downright shame, if not very close to a crime, that children (and adults, too) are subjected to such fattening and low-quality foods each and every morning.

- **You don't need breakfast to enhance your productivity.** Cereal companies and other such peddlers of breakfast foods like to say that if you skip breakfast, you won't get the necessary energy you need, and your productivity will suffer. This is all wrong. Chapter 2 discusses how fasting works to boost energy and productivity, which explains another reason why you don't need breakfast. What's doubly misleading, however, is that breakfast is in no way superior to fasting for energy, but in most cases, far inferior.

When you start your day with a bowl of sugar, which really is what most breakfast cereals are, you've set yourself up to experience turbulent blood sugar and an eventual crash. Remember, sugary foods spike blood sugar and insulin levels. And although you may get a quick surge of energy from the sugar at first, the end result, which is never far to follow, is invariably a sharp and unpleasant decline in energy.

Many food companies peddling breakfast cereals also want you to believe that the human body is a machine, and that without fuel in the morning it can't run properly. This is false. The human body is a biological organism, not a machine. You body doesn't need to be fed in the morning to run properly, because your body will still have in it plenty of energy reserves left over from the previous day of eating, and secondly, not eating allows your body to tap into stored body fat for a continuous stream of energy as well as enter into a natural and necessary state of detoxification.

If you're not entirely ready to give up breakfast, that's fine. Micro-fasting may not be the right fasting option for you. Check out the other chapters in Part II for other options. When you do eat breakfast, make sure it's worthwhile, and follow the same general guidelines as you would for all your other meals — start with protein and fibrous veggies, move onto healthy fats, and finish with more dense carbohydrate sources. An omelet with spinach and tomatoes would be a great choice. But again, the fasting benefits to be had from going without breakfast are simply too good to be ignored, and, too easy to take advantage of — really, all you have to do is push your first meal back a couple of hours!

Including Micro-Fasting in Your Life

If you're ready to begin to micro-fast, you may be curious about how you go about doing so. When you start, consider micro-fasting every day. Although you don't necessarily have to, from our experience, most people's adherence tends to improve when they micro-fast every day. That is, most people seem to have an easier time doing away with breakfast altogether and creating a new habit than they do when they just cut it out a couple days of the week.

Feel free to experiment with micro-fasting and see what works for you. If micro-fasting every day sounds like too much at first, work your way up gradually. Start with two to three days a week, and once you are comfortable with that, add another day every week or every other week. If you're going to implement micro-fasting, implement it at least two to three days a week.

Micro-fasting is about restricting the amount of time you eat throughout the day. In other words, you're simply compressing your daily food intake into an eight-hour window. This eight-hour window isn't an arbitrary number. Most of the benefits of fasting have been shown to occur within the first 16 hours.

(You may even want to shrink the fasting window to more than 16 hours. If so, check out the Warrior Diet in Chapter 7.) If you're ready to micro-fast, the following sections are the hands-on pieces that you need to get started. Here we discuss the ideal times when you can eat and what you can eat.

Identifying the ideal times to eat

Most people who practice micro-fasting say that 16 hours of fasting feels just right — you get hungry, but not too hungry. The peskiest part about micro-fasting, however, is identifying the ideal times to eat, more specifically, where to place your eight-hour eating window.

Most of the time, your first meal when micro-fasting happens sometime between noon and 2 p.m. To be successful, however, we recommend that you stick to a regular schedule. For example, if you stop eating at 8 p.m., you may start eating again each day around noon, which is a great schedule to live by. So in essence you eat from noon and 8 p.m. and fast from 8 p.m. to noon the next day.

Of course, you can play with micro-fasting a little bit. If you'd prefer to stop eating later, say around 9 p.m., then you simply move your eating window back an hour to 1 p.m. So long as you maintain the ratio of 16 hours of fasting to 8 hours of eating, you can be successful.

For your convenience, here are the five most popular eight-hour eating window schedules:

- ✔ 10 a.m. to 6 p.m.
- ✔ 11 a.m. to 7 p.m.
- ✔ 12 noon to 8 p.m.
- ✔ 1 to 9 p.m.
- ✔ 2 to 10 p.m.

Check out the last section in this chapter, "Diving Into Micro-Fasting — One Day" for an example of how you can apply micro-fasting to your life.

There are no hard rules to the eight hours that you eat. Our best advice is to make it work with your schedule. Don't make micro-fasting any more difficult than it needs to be. Place your eight-hour eating window where it's going to be most convenient for you. That is, make micro-fasting work with you, not you for it.

Recognizing what you can eat

The food you consume during the eight hours, how you choose to consume it, and how much you choose to consume greatly affect the effectiveness of your fasts. Fasting for 16 hours doesn't grant you permission to binge for the remaining eight.

Fasting works primarily by creating a caloric deficit. If you fast for 16 hours and then overcompensate the remaining eight, you're negating one of the primary benefits of fasting. So take our simple advice on what you can eat: Eat normally during your eight-hour window; in other words, eat only as much as you need to feel satisfied and not a smidgen more.

When eating, make sure you focus on quality over quantity. The quality of the food you put in your body is just as important as how much you consume. Furthermore, quantity dictates your weight, whereas the food quality impacts your overall health.

For what you eat, we again recommend the Paleo Diet, which simplifies making good food choices, because it focuses on eating foods that have the highest nutrient-to-calorie ratio, and eliminates all processed junk foods. Refer to Chapter 8 for what you can eat on the Paleo Diet and what you should eat when you're micro-fasting.

In addition, here a few more quick rules for eating during the eight-hour window:

- ✔ **Make your first meal your biggest meal.** Coming off your fast, ensure that your first meal is your biggest meal, especially if you just worked out. Fasting increases *assimilative capacity,* or how much food your body can process efficiently at one time. So yes, you can get away with eating a slightly larger meal than usual coming off a fast and not have to worry about storing excess body fat, as long as you don't completely overdo it.

- ✔ **Eat until you're satisfied, not stuffed.** A popular publication recently wrote an article on micro-fasting that misled people into thinking that they could eat whatever they wanted, as long as they kept their eating within an eight-hour window. This article was wrong. If something sounds too good to be true, it probably is. You want to eat sensibly throughout the eight hours, which means you eat healthful foods and only as much as you need to feel satisfied, not full, stuffed, or bloated.

- ✔ **Fill up on protein and veggies first.** Make your calories count, so fill up on the good stuff first — the stuff that has the highest nutrient-to-calorie ratio. In almost all cases, that stuff includes protein sources, such as fish, meat, and poultry, and fibrous vegetables, such as broccoli, kale, and cauliflower. From there you can move onto more complex carbohydrates, such as fruits and/or sweet potatoes.

✔ **Eat when you're hungry and don't eat when you're not hungry.** The eight-hour eating window doesn't mean that you should spend the entire eight hours eating. You want to eat when you're hungry and not eat when you're not hungry with a strong emphasis on the latter.

Space your meals out as much as possible to prevent overeating and to not overtax the digestive system. For example, having two meals four hours apart or something close to that is better than having one meal every hour.

The same foods you shouldn't eat when intermittent fasting also apply to micro-fasting. Check out Chapter 4 for a list of foods to avoid.

Timing Your Exercise with Micro-Fasting

Exercise is a critical factor for biological growth and rejuvenation. Engaging regularly in physical activity, especially bouts of short and intense exercise, is something everyone should do, no matter whether they're fasting or not. Specifically, integrating micro-fasting with your exercise plan can help you create the ultimate weapon to combat obesity, aging, and illness.

When micro-fasting, you should work out at the end of your 16-hour fast, so that immediately upon completion of your workout or soon thereafter, you can resume eating. Everyone ought to engage regularly in physical activity, especially bouts of short and intense exercise. Chapter 12 helps you to construct an exercise program, but for a more comprehensive exercise plan, refer to our book, *Paleo Workouts For Dummies* (John Wiley & Sons, Inc.).

Timing your exercise at the end of your micro-fast can give you a couple very important benefits:

✔ Fasting actually amplifies the effects of exercise. Chapters 2 and 11 provide more specific information.

✔ When you work out at the end of your fast, you can be sure that your first meal after your fast — which should also be your largest meal — is going toward repairing and building lean muscle tissue, and not being stored as body fat (as long as you don't overdo it, by eating a truly preposterous amount of food).

Try to get some form of exercise before every meal, because doing so helps to allocate nutrition to your muscles rather than body fat. Even a very brief workout — no more than five minutes — is enough to ensure that your muscles get priority. But there's a catch: The workout has to be relatively intense. Short lived, but intense. Refer to the later section "Diving Into Micro-Fasting — One Day" for an example of how to incorporate micro-fasting into your daily life.

Knowing What Types of Exercise Are Best When You're Micro-Fasting

You want to select certain types of exercise that give you the best results when you're micro-fasting. Some are better than others, and we discuss a couple of the really important ones that you should include in your workout regimen in these sections.

Here we explain why a combination of sprinting and heavy lifting (along with micro-fasting) can give you the results you want. For example, aim for 10 to 15 minutes of sprints combined with 15 to 20 minutes of heavy lifting, with a focus on the big compound movements such as squats, dead lifts, and pull-ups (all of which we discuss in Chapter 12) followed by 20 to 30 minutes of brisk walking to get the most out of your fasting periods.

Make sure you never begin an intense exercise program without your doctor's approval and a proper understanding of good form and exercise technique. Loading weight onto poor form is an impending disaster. It isn't a matter of if something is going to go wrong, but when. If you're unsure as to how to get started, or as to what the proper form for many exercise techniques should be, you can reference our book *Paleo Workouts For Dummies* (John Wiley & Sons, Inc.).

Sprinting

One of the best forms of intense exercise for blasting fat and building muscle is sprinting. When in a pinch, running 15 to 20 minutes of sprints at the end of your fast is a great way to get in your intense exercise for the day.

And no need to overcomplicate the matter, either. When it comes to sprinting, pick a distance that provides a good challenge but also allows you to be successful; you don't want the distance to be so long that your sprint turns into a jog. Be sure to rest as long as you need between sets of sprints until you feel fresh enough to do it again. Although this advice of taking your time may at first seem like a bit of a contradiction when it comes to sprinting, it's not. Sprinting is about expressing power, grace, and control. If you try to do too much too quickly, you'll express none of those things.

For example, sprint 50 meters, rest for one minute, sprint 100 meters, rest for two minutes, sprint 50 meters, rest for one minute, and so on for the total 15 to 20 minutes.

Sprinting involves super high-velocity muscular contractions, meaning that you had better be properly warmed up before you start sprinting. To warm up, always take the time to prep the body for the rigors of intense exercise with stretching, light movement, and a few warm-up sets of whatever you happen to be doing that day. With sprinting, warm up with a few sets of *strides* — which is a run that is somewhere between the intensity of a jog and a sprint.

Take at least 5 to 10 minutes to perform some light strides as well as another 5 to 10 minutes to perform some general stretching (such as a standing toe touch, performed with locked knees and a flat back) and foam rolling (which is a piece of equipment used to create supple muscle tissue).

Lifting heavy

Lifting heavy items is another important aspect of exercise when micro-fasting. Strength, loosely speaking, is the ability to generate tension in your muscles (which is what makes them contract). The only true way to increase strength is to increase tension in the muscles, and the only way to increase tension in the muscles is to lift more weight, lift the same weight with more speed, or a combination of the two. Chapter 11 focuses more on building strength by lifting.

As a result, in order for exercise to be intense enough to elicit muscular growth and rejuvenation, it needs to involve either a form of heavy strength training (heavy lifting), power training (fast lifting), or a combination of the two. Moderate-intensity aerobic activity, on the other hand, doesn't produce this effect, because it lacks the appropriate amount of intensity.

Our point is that you must not be afraid to lift heavy things. You do want to get the most out of your fasting and exercise program, right? *Heavy* is a relative term. What might be heavy for you, might not be heavy for us, and might not be heavy to a power lifter. As a general rule, if you can lift something for more than five to eight repetitions, then it's not heavy.

Although low-intensity aerobic activity, such as brisk walking, is very good for you and can help to boost many of the positive effects of fasting, research has shown that prolonged bouts of moderate-intensity aerobic activity, such as excessive amounts of jogging or cycling, may do more harm than good due to chronically elevated *cortisol* (that's your stress hormone), inflammation, and oxidative damage to cells. We suggest that you keep your aerobic work lower intensity (walking and hiking), or if you really enjoy moderate-intensity aerobic activity, just be sure not to overdo it (30 to 40 minutes, two to three days per week is more than enough in most cases).

Diving Into Micro-Fasting — One Day

This section provides an easy model to follow if you're seriously considering micro-fasting. Here we walk you through a day of micro-fasting, starting with the morning fasting routine, working through an intense exercise regimen, and finishing up with an eating window.

For the sake of convenience, we assume that you stopped eating the night before at approximately 8 p.m.

Here is what your day may look like if you're fasting:

6 a.m. You wake up, roll out of bed, and brew a fresh cup of organic green tea.

Light stimulants, such as organic green tea, pu-erh tea, black tea, and coffee are all permitted during a fast, as long as you don't put anything else into them, and as long as you don't overdo drinking them (one to two cups is more than enough) because they can help boost the positive effects of fasting, particularly fat burning.

7 a.m. You start your day with a brisk, 30-minute fasted walk outdoors.

When fasting — and even when not fasting — try to start your day with some form of light, fun activity to help naturally energize your mind and body. In conjunction with some green tea, it can also help to boost the fat-burning effects of fasting. Our first recommendation is brisk walking or hiking outdoors. Refer to the earlier section, "Timing Your Exercise with Micro-Fasting" for more information.

11: a.m. You begin your intense exercise routine (you can do this on your lunch break at work). After properly warming up, you do sprints for 15 minutes and lift heavy weights at a relatively high intensity for another 15 minutes. To cool down, you go for another brisk, 30-minute walk outdoors.

Noon You enjoy your first meal. You can opt for a spinach and salmon salad (spinach, salmon, cucumbers, tomatoes, extra-virgin olive oil, and balsamic vinegar). You can wash it down with clean, cool water, and then satisfy your sweet tooth with a handful or two of blueberries.

Start all your meals with protein, fats, and veggies, such as the spinach and salmon, before moving onto the more dense and/or sweet carbohydrates, such as the blueberries.

3 p.m. You're hungry again, so you fix another meal. This time you can eat exactly the same meal as before. It's actually a good practice, as well as convenient, to eat many of the same things over and over again. To be candid, a good diet is mostly a boring and repetitious one!

If it's the weekend or you're working from home, you can make an omelet with three eggs, spinach, onions, tomatoes, and peppers. You wash it down with a nice big glass of clean, cool water; this time, squeeze some fresh lemon into it.

6 p.m. Hunger strikes again! You eat a grass-fed steak with a generous side of asparagus and a small side salad, all brushed with extra-virgin olive oil. What's great about micro-fasting is that you still get to engage in the most social meal of the day — dinner! So this is where you can finally sit down and eat with your family.

7:30 p.m. Still a little hungry, you want one more meal before calling it a day. To keep it simple, you eat a handful of cashew nuts, a handful of mixed berries, and a few pieces of leftover turkey from the night before. You finish eating by 8 p.m., so your fast has to last until noon the next day.

10:30 p.m. Head to bed and aim for getting at least eight hours of sleep. Check out Chapter 13 for other ways you can improve your quality of life when fasting.

Make your last meal of the day a higher fat, lower carb meal, because fat helps promote sleep. A spoonful of almond or cashew butter is a great snack. As a general rule, stick just to nuts and meat for a good night's sleep. This example can show you how simple micro-fasting can be and that you don't need to make the practice unnecessarily complicated or difficult. When your eating window rolls around, eat whenever you're hungry; just stop eating when you're not hungry!

Chapter 7

Eating One Meal a Day: The Warrior Diet

*N*ot all fasting methods require that you completely abstain from eating during your fast. For example, although the 5:2 Diet, which we discuss in Chapter 5, necessitates undereating for an entire 24 hours, the Warrior Diet delineates the day into periods of undereating and overeating, which means you restrict what foods you can eat during the daytime, and at night you're able to enjoy a full, hearty meal. With the Warrior Diet, you don't fast just one or two times a week. Instead, you consistently engage in modified fasting every day. *Remember:* Fasting is part of an overall healthy lifestyle change, and the Warrior Diet is no exception to that.

This chapter explains exactly what the Warrior Diet is, from your daily period of undereating to the hours in which you overeat at night, and the pros and cons associated with this new lifestyle change. We also point out some foods that you can eat during the day and when undereating stops and the evening feast begins.

Explaining What the Warrior Diet Is: No Swords or Shields Required

The Warrior Diet is a modified fasting regimen where you don't completely restrict all calories — in liquid form or solid form — during your fast. The restriction focuses on consuming a small amount of food for most of the day and then eating as much as you want for several hours each evening.

The Warrior Diet is based on the premise that ancient people, who were fitter, healthier, and leaner than their modern counterparts, followed a daily regimen that included snacking only on healthful foods during the hours in which they completed most of their physical labor. They then reaped the fruits of that labor with a larger meal, recreation, and rest in the evening hours.

Although the term *warrior* may denote an overtly masculine character or a person whose job description vastly differs from your own, don't be mistaken. In reference to the Warrior Diet, *warrior* signifies a modern warrior, one who has decided that he or she is ready to make a return to instinctual eating, namely undereating and overeating, and tap into the many health benefits inherent in the warrior lifestyle. (We explain the concepts of overeating and undereating in the next section.)

Everything in nature is cyclical — from sunrises and sunsets to ocean tides to even human activities, such as sleeping and eating. The Warrior Diet is no exception, and it fits very well in the cycle of nature. Sometimes you eat very little. Sometimes you eat a lot. But at the end of the day (quite literally), it all gets balanced out. In other words, micro-periods of famine and feast inherently are built into each day.

Modeling your diet after ancient civilizations

Some ancient peoples, such as the Greeks and Romans, understood cyclical food consumption. They ate sparingly during the daytime hours and feasted together at night. They were also hardened warriors, lean, able-bodied, and mentally alert. They fought, they conquered, and they created great works of art, philosophy, and literature. We agree that people are only as capable as the food they put in their bodies and the way they go about eating that food. The Greeks and Romans were mightily capable.

However, if you look at the ancient Egyptians, you see something else entirely. The Egyptians of 3,000 or more years ago followed a diet and lifestyle similar to the typical ones of today. They were more sedentary. They ate grains and sweets, and they ate often, following the frequent feeding method that is so often touted in modern-day health and fitness magazines as the only way to "keep the metabolic fires burning."

And in the ancient Egyptian culture you can see what are described as the first known cases of diabetes, cancer, and metabolic syndrome — the very same diseases that run rampant in the modern world. We would be remiss to think that this similarity is merely coincidental, that what we as humans eat and how we eat doesn't directly affect our health and appearance.

The Warrior Diet aims to bring back the diet and nutrition styles of the ancient Greeks and Romans. It aims to nix the "eat often and eat at predetermined times" school of thought and return, instead, to eating by instinct. It may take time to regain those instincts, but by practicing the Warrior Diet, they will undoubtedly return.

Comparing Undereating and Overeating

Everything is cyclical, including your eating patterns. If you adhere to your natural eating patterns, then the Warrior Diet suggests that you must eat sparingly throughout the day and feast at night.

The human body has three major divisions of the nervous system, two of which you can directly affect by fasting:

- The *sympathetic* nervous system regulates the *fight or flight response*, which refers to activities that occur while the body is under stress (both everyday stress and abnormal stresses) and that keep your internal organs functioning properly.

- The *parasympathetic* system controls the body's *rest and digest* functions, which refers to the activities that occur when your body is at rest, such as digestion, sleep, and sexual arousal.

In other words, you should be fully within the sympathetic system during active daytime hours and in the parasympathetic system in the evening. Fasting is one of the most effective ways to ensure that these two systems are kept separate, as they naturally should be. On the Warrior Diet, you keep the two systems separated by undereating during the day and overeating in the evening hours.

But what undereating and overeating mean can be a little confusing, especially because so many of the popular diets today claim that you mustn't overeat and you certainly shouldn't eat too close to bedtime. Overeating paired with undereating is actually extremely effective for fat loss and building lean muscle mass. These sections help make sense of undereating and overeating so you have a better idea how the Warrior Diet works.

Tackling undereating and what you can eat during this phase

Undereating is the phase of the Warrior Diet that takes up most of day. You simply don't eat as much as you normally would during the daytime hours. You're naturally most active during these daytime hours, whether that activity is physical or mental.

During this undereating phase, the time when you restrict how much food you eat, you allow your body to give less energy toward digestive processes and relegate more energy to processes that will allow it to detoxify and cleanse itself, as well as burn fat, stabilize insulin levels, and promote the release of growth hormones. These benefits are similar to those benefits that you would encounter with any of the fasting methods described in this book. In general, fasting, whether true fasting or modified fasting such as the Warrior Diet or the 5:2 Diet (see Chapter 5), can have a phenomenal and positive impact on your health.

During the undereating phase, you eat and/or drink only fresh, raw produce and some light protein. Appropriate food and drink choices for the undereating phase might include the following:

- Black coffee or tea
- Unsweetened herbal tea
- Unsweetened coconut water
- Water
- Juice made from fresh raw vegetables and fruits
- Homemade broths that are free of monosodium glutamate (MSG), excessive salt, and hydrogenated oils
- Small servings of plain yogurt or kefir, or one to two eggs
- 16 ounces or less of all-natural whey protein shakes (whey mixed with water)
- Raw fruits or vegetables, such as a handful of berries, carrot sticks, or a grapefruit

Fresh is a description placed on many pre-packaged food products, particularly juice. And in the case of juice, the designation means that the juice wasn't made from concentrate. On the Warrior Diet, fresh juice means *really* fresh, which means that you should only drink those juices made before your eyes in a juicer or blender, not something that came in a bottle or jar.

If you're just starting on the Warrior Diet and are feeling deprived or just need some time to adapt to undereating, then you may also add a small handful of raw or dry roasted nuts, such as walnuts, almonds, or Brazil nuts.

While you're undereating during the day, consume only small servings of any calorie-containing foods or drinks. Remember that the goal of the undereating phase is to not eat a lot. You must exercise restraint during these daytime hours. Although doing so may seem quite difficult at first, you'll find that the longer you adhere to the Warrior Diet (or any fasting method, for that matter), the easier it will be to keep calorie intake to a minimum.

No matter how healthy you eat, getting all the essential vitamins, minerals, and other nutrients your body needs not only to function, but also to function optimally, can still be a challenge. Consider taking a high-quality multivitamin, probiotics, and/or fish oil to ensure you're getting everything you need on a regular basis.

Examining the overeating phase with common sense

Overeating on the Warrior Diet means just what you would expect. You eat more than you normally would, but only in the evening at your one meal. With overeating, you don't count calories, feel guilty eating high fat (but healthy) foods, or portion foods to ensure that you receive the appropriate fat, carbohydrates, and protein. Overeating simply means that you eat — starting with foods like a green salad and then moving to proteins, fruit and/or cooked veggies, denser carbohydrates, and/or healthy fats — until you feel full. You can usually tell that you're reaching the point of being full and satisfied when you start to feel more thirsty than hungry.

This concept of overeating means that you eat in an instinctual manner. Do you think that the Paleolithic human wondered about how many grams of fat he or she was eating in a day? Or what the protein-to-carb ratio in a given meal was? No, the ancient human feasted at the end of the long day and enjoyed that feast sans guilt. The Warrior Diet calls for a return to this healthier concept of overeating.

Overeating is okay on the Warrior Diet because you're overeating on healthy foods, not the typical junk that packs on fat and promotes disease. But you may be thinking that a calorie is a calorie. Much of the other diet advice you've heard throughout your life, just like this adage, isn't true.

When you overeat after fasting, your body is primed to use the calories and nutrients that you consume in a much more effective manner. Fat cells are released into the bloodstream and used up, nutrients assimilate into the body at a faster rate, greater amounts of lean muscle mass are built, secretions of your growth and other hormones increase (including *dopamine,* that "happy feeling" hormone), and body tissue is repaired.

A 2003 study on mice showed that those mice that were put on a fasting regimen combined with overeating, such as the regimen promoted in the Warrior Diet, saw a phenomenal increase in their overall health. Aging seemed to have been reversed. Diabetes disappeared. Cells repaired. And life span increased.

You may think of overeating as binging, gorging, and in general being a pig. Because of the various — and oftentimes, false — advice you may have heard over the years from well-meaning friends and family and by mainstream diet and exercise magazines, books, and blogs, you may believe that overeating will ultimately make you fail at reaching your fitness goals. Overeating on the Warrior Diet isn't about pigging out on ice cream, chicken fingers, pizza, burgers, and beer. Rather you simply eat healthful foods until you're full and satisfied. You eat enough to refuel the tank, so to speak, and don't feel guilty about it later.

So don't get caught up in the term "overeating." And don't feel guilty about it. Just remember that it isn't a free-for-all. You can overeat in a perfectly healthy way. You just want to make healthful food choices. Check out the later section, "Knowing what you can eat for your one meal" for what foods you should strive to eat in your one nightly meal.

Looking at the Power of Feast and Famine

The idea of feast and famine is one that has been part of humanity since ancient times and one that has been hard-wired into your DNA to have some pretty spectacular benefits. That doesn't mean, however, that, out of all the fasting methods discussed in this book, the Warrior Diet is the best fit for you. In these sections, we uncover the advantages and disadvantages of the Warrior Diet.

Perusing the pros of the Warrior Diet

Some of the advantages of the Warrior Diet include the following:

- ✔ You have the ability to eat (although lightly) throughout the day.
- ✔ It boosts metabolism.
- ✔ You have the freedom to overeat and enjoy food without the typical diet guilt.
- ✔ You see an improvement in overall health — from vitality to virility.
- ✔ Your lean muscle mass increases.
- ✔ You return to instinctive and healthy eating patterns.
- ✔ It slows the aging process.

As with the other fasting methods outlined in this book, the Warrior Diet is free of extraneous supplements or diet pills, and you don't have to work through any complicated formulas to figure out what you can or can't eat.

Discussing the disadvantages of the Warrior Diet

The Warrior Diet is a fasting method that truly embodies the idea of a lifestyle overhaul. For some people, this challenge may be too much at first.

The Warrior Diet may also be challenging because the undereating period that you engage in each day is longer than the fasting time in, say, the micro-fasting method in Chapter 6. And though you do eat a very hearty meal while adhering to the Warrior Diet, you only get to eat one meal a day.

You may want to experiment with whether or not adhering to a modified fasting program, such as the Warrior Diet, would actually be more difficult for you than simply cutting out food and calorie-laden drinks altogether. Some people find that eating lightly, rather than completely abstaining, makes the fast harder to get through.

Consuming Just One Meal a Day

The Warrior Diet is derived from the concept that traditional societies, those whose people were lean, strong, and physically and mentally tough — those who embodied the *warrior spirit* — only ate one meal a day. Although the technologies of today all but eliminate the basic physical endeavors, you can return to this primal living by adhering to the same kind of eating strategy.

The hormonal and physical benefits of fasting in this warrior fashion (or undereating throughout the day and overeating at night) are incredible, from gaining strength and muscle to finally getting rid of stubborn body fat to detoxifying your body to boosting virility. The Warrior Diet's concept of eating one meal a day keeps your body in warrior mode, making you mentally alert and physically lean and muscular.

The following sections discuss exactly how you should approach the Warrior Diet and eating only one meal a day, as well as how to know when to stop eating and when to start.

Knowing what you can eat for your one meal

The foods that you can eat during the undereating phase are different from those foods that you can consume during the nightly overeating phase, although the guidelines for both phases follow similar rules. Here are some general guidelines to follow on the Warrior Diet so you know what to eat in your evening meal. You can also check out Chapter 8 for specific food suggestions.

✔ **Choose fresh, natural, and wholesome foods.** These foods, particularly raw vegetables, are typically subtle in taste, meaning they won't overpower your taste buds with processed sugar, refined fats, salt, or artificial flavorings. In this sense, the Paleo Diet is a perfect complement to the Warrior Diet method of fasting. (Refer to Chapter 8 for more on the ins and outs of the Paleo Diet.)

Although you won't just be eating raw veggies on the Warrior Diet, you should start there. Focus on eating subtle-tasting foods and then move onto protein, then cooked vegetables, and finally round out your meal with either carbohydrate-rich foods, such as fruits and sweet potatoes, or the occasional dessert or fat-rich foods, such as nuts, nut butters, or high-fat desserts.

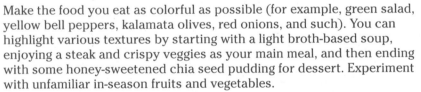

Make the food you eat as colorful as possible (for example, green salad, yellow bell peppers, kalamata olives, red onions, and such). You can highlight various textures by starting with a light broth-based soup, enjoying a steak and crispy veggies as your main meal, and then ending with some honey-sweetened chia seed pudding for dessert. Experiment with unfamiliar in-season fruits and vegetables.

✔ **Start with subtle-tasting foods.** In the Standard American Diet (SAD) of today, *subtle-tasting* foods are unfortunately uncommon. If you go to any restaurant, the first thing you'll see set in front of you is a basket of bread rolls made from heavily processed flour or tortilla chips fried in vegetable oil. However, the best and healthiest choices include a large green salad topped with tomatoes, onions, carrots, bell peppers, and a simple olive oil and vinegar dressing.

✔ **Choose between a meal of protein paired with carbohydrate-rich foods or a meal of protein and fat-rich foods.** Selecting one of these two options maximizes your body's ability to absorb nutrients, burn calories, and keep everything running smoothly. If you go with the first option, pick a lean protein with carbohydrates, such as sweet potatoes. You can also go with a meal of protein and fat-rich foods, such as nuts and seeds. Try to alternate those carb-heavy and fat-heavy meals.

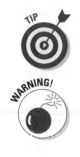

One method to help you not only opt for the best food choices but to also keep you interested and excited in the food you're eating is to include as many different flavors, textures, colors, and aromas as you can within your nightly meal.

✔ **Watch out for store-bought dressings.** If you prepare your own foods, then you're in direct control as to what actually goes into the food you eat. It takes as little time to drizzle extra-virgin olive oil and balsamic vinegar on a salad as it does to pour ready-made dressings on it. Beware of those store-bought dressings. Even if they seem innocuous enough (such as a bottle of balsamic vinaigrette), those products can have loads of extraneous ingredients, from preservatives to sugar. Play it safe — and healthy — and make your own. We include dressings in a few of the salad recipes in Chapters 9 and 10.

Otherwise you have few restrictions. You can eat as much as you want during your one nightly meal. Although this concept of healthful overeating may feel foreign or guilt-inducing, you'll find that the longer you practice the Warrior Diet, the more attuned to your body you'll become, meaning you'll instinctively know when to stop eating and what it feels like to be truly full and satisfied.

Play, invent, and use your imagination. Meal preparation is an inherently creative process. There's no reason or excuse to get bored preparing and eating healthy foods.

Just because you've successfully completed a fast or a string of fasting days, whether or not you are adhering to the Warrior Diet, don't celebrate by derailing your nutrition. The Warrior Diet helps detoxify your body so don't fall into the trap of putting toxins back in with sweet treats, refined sugar, and processed grains.

Following important eating guidelines

When adhering to the Warrior Diet, the undereating phase lasts the vast majority of the day — about 20 hours — whereas the overeating phase that occurs in the evening lasts the remaining four hours.

Although you can think of the four hours as one large meal, aim to break up the various meal components (subtle-tasting greens, protein, veggies, and fruits/dessert) as you see fit across that time period. Don't worry about how much you're eating, instead listen to your body and only eat to satiety.

How you divide your fasting day is up to you. Just keep the following overall guidelines to help ensure that you complete a successful fast:

Drink plenty of quality water

The undereating phase doesn't have any limits on water or other noncaloric beverages. So go for it and drink as much filtered water as you want. You should drink plenty of *filtered* water. Living in the modern world, you may think that water that comes from the tap is perfectly safe to drink. We would agree, but oftentimes drinking tap water actually isn't safe.

We suggest that you aim to consume more than the standard eight-glasses-a-day recommendation. In fact, eight glasses of eight ounces each (totaling 64 ounces) should be the bare minimum, especially on days when you're also exercising (which you should be doing, at least in some form, whether it be walking or metabolic conditioning, each day). Fasting helps detoxify the body, and drinking water helps flush those toxins out of your system.

Drinking filtered water is especially important because tap water can contain more than a thousand toxins, including chlorine, fluoride, lead, mercury, nitrates, pesticides, and many more. A 2008 study also found prescription medications, from antidepressants to sex hormones, in the tap water that more than 40 million Americans drink on a regular basis. Although at any given time, the concentration of such contaminants is most likely quite low, over the span of your life, they build up in the system and can contribute to some awful diseases.

Take chlorine, for instance. The accumulation of chlorine in your body can cause heart and circulatory diseases and can kill the good bacteria in the digestive tract that you need to maintain a healthy digestion. (Probiotics are often touted as a good supplement to aid in digestion. However, if you're taking probiotics and drinking tap water, you may very well be flushing money down the toilet.)

To ensure that you're drinking filtered water, hook a carbon-based filter to your sink, so you're drinking and cooking only with the water that gets filtered through it. Just make sure you drink plenty of it.

Understanding protein's role during the undereating and overeating stages

With solid foods, during the undereating phase, you can have small servings of protein, such as one or two boiled eggs, a scant cup of kefir or yogurt, and a protein shake made from all-natural whey or milk protein. If you're really in need of a caloric boost, a small handful of raw or sprouted unsalted nuts is okay. Also, feel free to enjoy raw vegetables and fruit, such as blueberries or carrots.

Despite the name, peanuts aren't nuts. They are legumes, like kidney beans or chickpeas. Stick to Brazil nuts, pistachios, walnuts, almonds, and so on. If you're extremely athletic and are burning thousands of calories a day in vigorous athletic activity, then you may need to eat more during the day in the way of carbohydrates, such as including a sweet potato in your under-eating phase. However, perhaps the best strategy, if possible, is to time those incredibly intense training sessions so that they come at the end of the undereating phase.

Some days you're just hungrier than others. Although the goal of the Warrior Diet is to restrict calories and undereat for most of the day, if you're feeling deprived or are adapting to a more intense training regimen, you may add in some extra carbs during the day. However, your best bet (should fat loss be your goal) is to opt for an extra-light protein-based meal instead.

At the end of the day, during your overeating phase, you can eat as much as you want at your only regular meal. Break your fast with raw veggies, protein, broth-base soups, fruit, cooked veggies, and from time to time dessert.

Realizing the truth about eating later in the day

No doubt that at some time or another you've read, heard, and maybe even believed that eating at night makes you fat and that you mustn't eat anything past a certain hour if you want to finally free yourself from the stubborn fat that clings to your body. The truth is that if you're eating healthy, wholesome, natural foods, and you fast or undereat for most of the day, eating at night won't make you fat and it won't keep extra weight on your body that refuses to come off.

The human body is meant to eat in the evening. Eating is an activity that the body understands to be part of the rest-and-digest phase of the day (refer to the earlier section, "Comparing Undereating and Overeating" for more information) and one that should be paired with other restorative and rejuvenating practices, such as relaxing on the couch, going for a quiet stroll, watching TV, and yes, sleeping and engaging in sexual activities.

If you've ever tried to go to sleep while hungry, you know it's nearly impossible because just as eating during the day can trigger feelings of sleepiness, not eating at night can keep you feeling alert and awake. In other words, you can confuse your body's nervous systems. Eating during the day can put your body into the rest-and-digest parasympathetic system, and not eating at night can make your body think that it needs to still be in the fight-or-fight sympathetic system.

When you gorge on fattening ice cream, fried foods, potato chips, and other packaged and processed foods, you'll put on weight, no matter what time of the day you consume them.

Part III

Your Launch Pad to Fasting: Your Kitchen and Recipes

Detoxifying with fruit and vegetable juices when fasting

Juicing is the process of extracting juice from fresh fruits and vegetables. It's beneficial because the juice from fresh fruits and vegetables is full of antioxidants, vitamins and minerals, and live enzymes (which makes the juice easy on the digestive system). Juicing is best used in conjunction with a controlled fast, such as the 5:2 Diet, the Warrior Diet, and micro-fasting, which allows for the light consumption of live foods throughout the day. Here are some powerful fruits and vegetables that you can experiment with. They're all low-glycemic and highly nutrient dense.

- Beets
- Berries (blueberries, blackberries, strawberries, raspberries)
- Broccoli
- Cabbage
- Carrot and ginger
- Cauliflower
- Cucumber
- Grapefruit
- Lemon
- Lime
- Spinach

When juicing, stick to the juice from fresh fruits and vegetables and not store-bought juices.

Go to www.dummies.com/extras/fastdiets for some bonus 500- and 600-calorie recipes.

In this part...

- Discover different cooking methods and food preparation techniques, such as broiling and sautéing, that can make your fasting lifestyle more effective and efficient.

- Peruse the simple kitchen equipment, such as a cutting board, knives, baking sheets, a colander, a food processor and/or blender, and other items that can make cooking and preparing your food easier.

- Examine some helpful tips for shopping for healthful foods you can eat during your nonfasting meals.

- Understand why processed foods, grains, and refined sugars are sabotaging your efforts to live a healthy life.

- Comprehend why eating fat doesn't make you fat and why all fats aren't created equal, including which fats you should include in your diet on a regular basis and which ones you should strictly avoid.

- For women, see how to build your own 500-calorie meal plan that is diverse, uncomplicated, easy-to-follow, and deprivation-free.

- For men, find out how to create — and stick to — a 600-calorie fasting meal plan that won't leave you feeling unsatisfied.

Chapter 8

Restocking Your Kitchen with Foods You Can Eat during Your Fast and Meals

. . . .

In This Chapter

▶ Beginning your fast the right way

▶ Introducing the foods to be consumed during your fasting eating window

▶ Embracing healthy and satisfying grain-free, dairy-free, non-inflammatory foods

▶ Discovering what foods to avoid

▶ Making healthy cooking choices

. . . .

*T*his chapter is about discovering the foods that work best for your body during your fasting *eating window* (the time when you can consume food when you're not actually fasting). They're all non-inflammatory and *hydrating-dense* (high nutrition relative to foods' calories), which provide the best raw materials to help your body function at a higher level. When your body is given the ability to recalibrate with these foods, you start losing fat naturally, your eyes brighten, and your skin glows. You begin to think more clearly, and your mood lifts. All these benefits are yours when you create a healthy internal environment and provide your body with sufficient nutrition.

Just think of it this way: Where there is waste, there is weight. Where there is deficiency, there is illness. Eating non-inflammatory, nutrient-rich foods is your answer to these situations. Your body fine-tunes and refines to a healthier state.

When your body isn't working hard to deal with what it doesn't need, it focuses on getting you more of what you do need. This is the premise behind fasting, and eating the right foods during your eating window. You get healthier, stronger, and leaner. When you begin to eat these foods, you'll be shocked by the way your body composition begins to change and your energy skyrockets.

If you're going to give yourself limited calories a few days a week (as with the 5:2 Diet in Chapter 5), then make them count by giving your body nutrient density. The best way to transition to a leaner, healthier, strong body is to give it the right raw material.

In this chapter, we help you discover the best foods for fueling your body during this time of caloric reduction, the foods that should be consumed during your fasting-eating window, and the foods that you should steer clear of — particularly when on a fasting schedule. In addition, we explain some healthy cooking methods and describe what you should be looking for in your food to find the top quality.

Including Items You Can Eat

Restocking your kitchen with all the best foods is where the real commitment begins. These sections identify the foods that can help you look and feel your best while fasting — or anytime.

Your ultimate goal when restocking your kitchen is to make sure you're getting nutrients in the highest amounts. Your body can handle eating small amounts of food beautifully when it's still getting what it needs in terms of nutrients. The tipping point of getting those nutrients is all about food quality. The higher the quality of food choices means the more nutrition that food will have. When selecting fasting foods, make sure that all the foods you choose are from *real food sources* (food that isn't made in a lab or processed in any way) with a focus on the best quality you can afford. That's it. You don't need any special pills or juices to get the best nutrition.

Focus your eating on quality meats, fish, seafood, and eggs; healthy fats and oils; vegetables and fruits; and nuts and seeds. They give your body the raw material it craves to be to be strong, lean, and healthy. All the processed, denatured foods, premade frozen foods, packaged foods, and sugary carbohydrates need to be kicked to the can! They only feed cravings and cause weight gain and disease.

You've likely spent a long time developing your eating habits, so breaking them and instituting new ones may take some time. The longer you've depended on sugary foods, the more difficult retraining your taste buds to recognize natural sweetness may be. Using healthful foods to fuel your body will go a long way in keeping you super lean and strong — for the long run. Fasting plus eating the approved eating window foods we discuss in these sections is pure magic!

Looking at what's behind those cravings

Keeping your foods simple, real, and unprocessed can even help you with your sugar cravings. When you have a craving, your body is usually looking for a quick burst of something to make it feel better. Often that something is a brain chemical called *serotonin*. This chemical affects mood, specifically happiness and well-being. The higher the levels of serotonin in your body the happier you feel.

When your serotonin levels drop, your body screams out for a change. It's looking for that "feel good" chemical to alter its brain chemistry. This chemical is one of the reasons so

many people are in the vicious cycle of eating sweets, processed foods, or a lot of carbohydrates. When people feel tired, depressed, or down, they look for something to make them feel good and change their state of mind, so they self-medicate with these foods.

When you feel those cravings come on, it may be because you're just having a bad day or are under a lot of stress, so be mindful of the *why* behind your sweet cravings. The best way to maintain your serotonin levels is to eat the foods that work best within your body and exercise.

Not having the money to purchase your desired food choices can sometimes be frustrating. Just know: You're still making monumental strides in getting lean and living long and strong when you take up the fasting principles we discuss in this book and eat the non-inflammatory foods we recommend. Just do the best you can and don't stress out (which is even worse for you than eating a lower quality food!). Use this book as a guide to help you do your best when making the most important choice you can make in your life — what you fuel your body with.

Power proteins

Protein builds you up. Growth and repair are protein's major roles; your body uses the protein you take in from foods to build cells, synthesize new proteins, and keep your tissues healthy. Eating adequate protein supports your physique and keeps you full for a long time.

Food quality is particularly important when dealing with protein. Getting the best quality proteins can provide you with tons of nutrition. Focus on knowing what to buy and start incorporating higher quality foods into your budget whenever you can. If you can't do the highest quality right now, just remember how much good you're doing your body getting rid of all the processed foods and eating more non-inflammatory foods.

Here's what's really awesome: Protein burns fat! When your body gets enough protein, you can increase the rate at which your metabolism burns calories. Your body requires more energy to break down protein because the protein isn't readily available to use for energy as carbohydrates are. This extra work your body has to do to efficiently use fat for fuel promotes fat burning.

The following sections identify some ideal proteins to eat during your fast or your eating window and help you figure out food labels to ensure you're consuming the best quality food.

Egg quality

Nailing down the quality of eggs is extra important because eggs are such a common protein. This list helps you decode labels when you're shopping for eggs:

- **Pasture raised:** Chickens can roam freely. Their diet consists of nutritious grasses and other plants and bugs.

- **Cage free:** These chickens aren't roaming around freely in the great outdoors. In other words, they're kept inside barns or warehouses with no access to the outdoors; they're allowed to roam only inside the barn or warehouse. The living conditions can vary greatly.

- **Certified organic:** Chickens are given organic feed, and no antibiotics, unless they're ill and require them. They must be uncaged and have some access to the outdoors. There is compliance through auditing.

- **Natural:** This label is somewhat sketchy because it means absolutely nothing. What it really means is the chicken is minimally processed.

- **Free range:** This label means the chicken has access to outdoors at least 51 percent of the time. There are no restrictions on what the birds are fed. Because this label isn't certified, there really is no way of knowing how long these chickens are roaming around outside.

- **Omega-3:** Chickens were fed fish oil or flaxseed, but who knows how much because it's not regulated.

- **United Egg Producers Certified:** This labeling is extremely misleading because it permits routine cruel and inhumane farm practices and caging. It has no value whatsoever.

- **Vegetarian:** This label means that hens are fed a diet free of animal byproducts, which is a bit nonsensical because chickens aren't vegetarians, so they aren't being fed what is actually a natural diet to them.

- **No antibiotics/No hormones:** This is more of a marketing ploy because if you're buying certified organic, Animal Welfare Approved, or Humane Certified eggs, neither antibiotics nor hormones are allowed anyway. Knowing the validity of the label is difficult because the term isn't regulated.

✔ **Animal Welfare Approved:** This label is a very high welfare standard, reserved mostly for family farms. The hens have continual access to shelter and pasture with no antibiotic use. This term is regulated.

✔ **Food Alliance Certified:** Hens are uncaged and have access to the outdoors. This label is also regulated.

✔ **American Humane Certified:** This label allows for cage confinement and cage-free systems. The problem though is there is no way of knowing which one you're getting — cage confined or cage free. If the hens are caged confined, the space the hens have is the size of a legal sheet of paper.

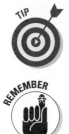

So many choices! So to ensure that you're getting the best eggs, we suggest you focus on buying eggs labeled organic, pasture-raised. Certified humane or Food Alliance Approved are assurances that the chicken were humanely and healthily raised.

Many people have eliminated eggs or egg yolks from their diets because of the risk of elevating their cholesterol levels. This is simply based on untrue and misguided information. In fact, studies show that dietary cholesterol has very little affect on blood cholesterol. Actually, the egg yolk contains *choline,* which is a natural fat transporter, keeping cholesterol out of the blood. Dietary cholesterol simply isn't a good indicator of heart disease. Eggs also contain vitamins B12 and D, riboflavin, and folate that may help prevent heart disease.

Meat quality

Meat obviously is a great source of protein. Here are some quality guidelines when selecting different types of meat:

✔ **Beef:** Selecting local, pasture-raised, grass-fed beef is your best choice. If you aren't purchasing organic, grass-fed, then be sure to choose lean cuts, and trim all visible fat off beef as well as drain all excess fat. Selecting mainstream, traditional, lean cuts with the visible fat trimmed is an okay choice.

✔ **Poultry:** The best cuts are organic, pasture-raised chicken or turkey that's also free of antibiotics and hormones. All cuts, including the tasty chicken livers, are good choices. If your chicken or turkey isn't organic and pastured, remove the skin prior to eating.

✔ **Pork products:** Focus on buying local, pasture-raised pork because you can avoid the hazards of the omega-6 fatty acids (inflammation-producing fats) found in factory-farmed pork. If you can't purchase at least organic, free-range pork, we suggest you avoid commercial pork and select another protein. US Wellness Meats is a fantastic resource at www. grasslandbeef.com/StoreFront.bok.

- ✔ **Lamb:** Pasture-raised, grass-fed cuts are healthy and laden with nutrients. The nutrient-dense organ meats are a great source of B12 and zinc as well, good for healing during your eating window.

- ✔ **Wild game:** All game including bison, goat, elk, venison, duck, wild boar, ostrich, and rabbit.

  Fish (tuna, salmon, sardines, mackerel, and so on), seafood, and shellfish: To find the healthiest, highest quality seafood, shellfish, and fish, look for *wild fish* (caught in the wild), *wild caught fish* (may have spent some time in a fish farm), or fish that was humanely harvested. For the ultimate guide, please refer to the Monterey Bay Aquarium's free list of the best seafood choices: www.montereybayaquarium.org/cr/cr_seafoodwatch/sfw_recommendations.aspx.

Most companies use very poor quality oils in their canned fish. You should also always check the labels for soy. Also, don't buy canned fish with anything but water added. It's best to just add the oil at home. Vital Choice (www.vitalchoice.com/shop/pc/home.asp) carries high-quality canned fish.

- ✔ **Deli meats, or chicken or turkey sausage:** These meats should be antibiotic and gluten-free with no nitrates or nitrites.

If you're on a strict budget and have to pick and choose where you spend any extras, we recommend you throw down the extra bucks on meat. Getting healthy meat on a budget is more difficult than finding other healthy conventional foods. If you buy conventional meats, make sure you chose the leanest cuts and trim all visible fats before cooking.

Ensuring that your beef is grass-fed and grass-finished

When you consume beef, you want to make sure your beef is completely grass-fed and grass-finished so you can thereby get all the healthy fats and nutrition from consuming the beef. Check to see that the cattle were fattened with grass only and not grain (usually corn) during the last 90 to 160 days before they were processed.

If the cattle eat grain during this 90- to 160-day finishing process, the levels of important nutrients like conjugated linoleic acid (CLA), which is a healthy fat that prevents many diseases such as cancer, heart disease, high blood pressure, inflammation, and more, are lower. This is a fat you actually want in your diet. Omega-3 (another wonderfully healthy fat that so many people are deficient in) decreases dramatically in the beef's animal tissues. Grain may be fed to cattle to fatten them up more quickly so they get to slaughter more quickly, but the nutrient profile isn't nearly as healthy in the grains as in the grass, which ultimately affects your health.

Nutrient-dense produce

Carbohydrates in the form of produce (fruits and vegetables) give you the fuel your body needs for bursts of energy. Whether you eat cookies or kale, your body transforms the carbohydrates into glucose. Your brain and your cells use this glucose for fuel for your daily activities, which means the quality of your health and how lean you become depends a great deal on what carbohydrates you choose to use as fuel.

You can compare it to fueling your car: The better the gas you use, the better your car will run, and the more you'll get out of it. Consuming healthier carbohydrates is particularly important when you're fasting, striving to get your body in a fat-burning mode, and training your body be an efficient fat burner long-term.

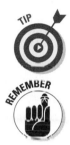

If you want to stay lean and healthy, you have to be savvy when it comes to carbohydrates. Where there is excess insulin, there is fat. As a result, knowing what carbs to eat is key in burning fat and feeling your best.

When choosing produce, think variety, color, and in-season whenever possible. Creating a meal with two vegetables is a great way to bring nutrients to your plate. Consider these options:

- ✔ **Leafy greens:** High in fiber, vitamins, and minerals, leafy greens are some of the best veggies to put on your plate. Try beet tops, bok choy, collard greens, kale, mustard greens, Napa cabbage, spinach, Swiss chard, and turnip greens.

- ✔ **Hearty vegetables:** Roasted, sautéed, or steamed, these veggies serve up plenty of flavor and nutrition. Dig into artichokes, asparagus, beets, broccoli, Brussels sprouts, cabbage, cauliflower, carrots, eggplant, fennel, onion, parsnips, spaghetti squash, summer squash, turnips, and zucchini.

- ✔ **Salad vegetables:** Fresh, crisp, and filling, a salad can be a meal in itself or a tantalizing side. Toss in alfalfa sprouts, arugula, bell peppers, celery, cucumber, jicama, lettuce (such as romaine, Boston, Bib, iceberg, escarole, or red leaf), mushrooms, radicchio, radishes, red cabbage, sunflower sprouts, tomatoes, and watercress.

- ✔ **Carb-dense vegetables:** These starchy and carbohydrate-dense vegetables play an important role in helping you recover from exercise and stress. Roast a batch of acorn squash, butternut squash, spaghetti squash, sweet potatoes, or yams. Toss some jicama, kohlrabi, or beets in a salad. You can even sauté some plantains for a yummy treat!

✔ **Approved legumes:** Although these vegetables are technically legumes, (legumes aren't one of the approved fasting window foods because they cause digestive distress for those people not accustomed to eating them), they include more pod than bean — and they're green! Snap into green beans, string beans, snap peas, snow peas, and wax beans.

Legumes are beans, peas, and lentils. With the exception of the approved legumes that we just mentioned, we suggest you pass on legumes to lose weight, perform better, and heal conditions. If you're a vegetarian and don't eat fish or eggs, you have to get some source of protein in your diet, so you can eat legumes. But for most people, legumes are a very starchy food, with not much protein, so you're getting a lot of starch, with small amounts of protein, which isn't good for your health. Also, most people find them very hard to digest and experience gut disturbances, such as bloating, after eating them. If you're looking to get fiber, fill your plate with some vegetables, and you'll be good to go.

✔ **Fresh herbs:** Leafy herbs like basil, cilantro, dill, garlic, ginger, mint, oregano, parsley, rosemary, and thyme add a big dose of flavor to any meal.

✔ **Fruits:** Eaten whole or in salads, raw or cooked, colorful fruits are a good source of vitamins and taste oh so sweet. Savor every bite, from apples to kiwi. Dark-colored fruits, such as blackberries, blueberries, strawberries, raspberries, cherries, and cranberries, are filled with antioxidants and low in natural sugars, which is why they're our favorites.

Satisfiingly sweet friuts you can eat include apples, apricots, bananas, blackberries, blueberries, cantaloupe, cherries, cranberries, dates, figs, grapefruits, grapes, honeydews, kiwis, kumquats, lemons, limes, mangos, nectarines, oranges, papayas, peaches, pomegranates, raspberries, strawberries, tangerines, tomatoes, and watermelons.

Eat dried fruits, which are high in sugar, in moderation. You can add them to stews, sautés, and vegetables to add texture and a hint of sweetness. Always check labels for preservatives and *sulfites,* preservatives that aren't healthy. They're commonly found in dried fruits. Also think of dried fruit as a natural sweetener and not as a food to aimlessly munch on.

With produce, your budget has a little more leeway. What's most important is that you just eat your vegetables. However, quality can make a difference with the nutrients and even reduce the toxins or pesticides that may be found in your produce. Ideally, you want to purchase local and organic vegetables and fruit. If your budget is tight, you can purchase mainstream. Just make sure you rinse the vegetables to remove any possible pesticides.

For a handy guide to show you what vegetables and fruits you can use conventional, check out the Environmental Working Groups Dirty Dozen and Clean 15 Guide list at www.ewg.org/foodnews/guide.

Comparing the types of fats

All this talk about healthy fats deserves a short explanation. Consider this your chemistry course on healthy fats. Types of healthy fats include the following:

✔ **Saturated fats:** They have single bonds only and contain mostly saturated fatty acids. Saturated fats are solid at room temperature and get harder when chilled. Good sources of saturated fats include coconut oil, coconut flakes, coconut milk, coconut butter, and organic clarified butter from grass-fed cows. (*Clarified butter* is the full butter fat that is left after the milk and the water have been removed from the butter, so even if you're lactose-intolerant, this type may be a good option for you.)

Researchers are finding more evidence that higher saturated fat intake does *not* increase the risk of developing heart disease. Not only are saturated fats powerful antiviral and antifungal agents and key players in immune health, but they can also do the following:

• Allow for proper nerve signaling

• Build stronger bones

• Fight autoimmune disease

• Lower (yes, lower!) cholesterol

• Ward off cancer

✔ **Monounsaturated fats:** *Monounsaturated fats* (MUFAs) contain one double bond and have mostly monounsaturated fatty acids. These fats are liquid at room temperature and get thicker when chilled. Good sources of this type of fat include olives (green or black), olive oil, avocado, avocado oil, macadamia nuts, macadamia oil, cashew nuts, cashew butter, and hazelnuts. MUFAs are super-healthy and fantastic on salads.

To use oils to boost immunity, figure out the *smoke point* of that oil — the point where the oil starts to break down and starts to burn or smoke. When the oil has reached this point, it becomes rancid and will derail your attempts to consume healthy fats. You can find a handy smoke point chart at www.goodeatsfanpage.com/collectedinfo/oilsmokepoints.htm.

✔ **Polyunsaturated fats:** *Polyunsaturated fats* (PUFAs) have more than one double bond and contain mostly polyunsaturated fatty acids. Polyunsaturated fats are liquid at room temperature and stay liquid when chilled. Good sources of polyunsaturated fats include almonds, almond butter, Brazil nuts, pistachios, pecans, chestnuts, walnuts, pumpkin seeds, sesame seeds, sunflower seeds, sunflower butter, and pine nuts.

PUFAs are just a bit higher in omega-6 ratios than MUFAs, so consume PUFAs in moderation. For example, avocado, which is a MUFA, has an omega-6 to omega-3 ratio of 12:1. Walnuts, which are PUFAs, have a ratio of 53:10.

Healthy fats

Understanding healthy fats and the value they have during your eating window is one of the most important principles you can discover in nutrition. Eating healthy fats actually helps you lose stored body fat for overall weightloss, protects you against heart disease, melts away inflammation, and aides in conditions like skin disorders, arthritis, high cholesterol, high triglycerides, diabetes, and depression. Healthy fats also make you feel fuller and satisfied. For instance, if you're fasting, having healthy fats the day before makes having a reduced caloric intake the day after much easier because you aren't hungry.

Healthy fats make all the structures and functions of your body flourish. You need them for hormone production and for the growth and development of the brain, immune system, nervous system, heart, and blood vessels. Healthy fats also make you look younger by nourishing the skin and giving it a beautiful sheen, making your hair shiny, diminishing wrinkles, and giving you a beautiful, healthy appearance.

We need to set the record straight on a couple of familiar assertions about fats:

✔ The key to a leaner body has nothing to do with a low-fat diet. In fact, to access stored fat in your body for energy, you need to consume fats in your meals so you can then burn stored fat for energy.

✔ Saturated fats aren't the cause of heart disease. Studies are revealing more and more that inflammation caused from all the processed oils (see the nearby sidebar for more information) and refined foods are the culprits of heart disease — not the healthy, good old, back-to-nature fats we explain in this section.

So what are healthy fats? Essential fats (omega-3 and omega-6 fatty acids) are healthy fats. (Refer to the nearby sidebar for more information about these two fatty acids.) Your body doesn't produce these fats on its own, so you must consume them in order to get the benefits. (Lucky for you, healthy fats make foods taste better and help you feel satisfied.) Including essential fats in your diet will definitely give you an edge in looking and feeling your best.

Finding balance with omega-6 and omega-3 fats

Omega-6 is one of two types of essential fatty acids. Omega-3 is its counterpart. A proper balance of these two types of fatty acids helps to keep chronic inflammation, which can lead to a whole host of health issues, including heart disease and cancer, at bay.

Fatty acids are essential to humans; the human body needs them but can't internally make them. You must supplement your diet by consuming both omega-3 and omega-6 fatty acids from various foods.

Research suggests that humans evolved to require a desirable ratio of omega-6 and omega-3 fatty acids, about a 1:1 ratio. However, in modern Western diets, that ratio is grossly out of whack. Think upwards of 15:1 or 16:1. Omega-6 fatty acids are rampant in many of the foods people eat today, including butter substitutes, grain fed animal products, canola oil, cottonseed oil, and soybeans, among other things. Omega-3 fatty acids, on the other hand, can be found in especially high concentrations in flax, algae, grass fed animal products, wild-caught salmon, mackerel, anchovy, and fish oil.

A 2008 study showed that there was an increased probability of people developing coronary heart disease, diabetes, arthritis, cancer, osteoporosis, mental illness, dry eye disease, and age-related macular degeneration if they consumed too much omega-6 and not enough omega-3 to offset it. Omega-3 fatty acid, on the other hand, helps circulation by naturally thinning the blood, lessening inflammation, supporting brain function (just as fasting does — talk about a triple whammy!), and even easing the symptoms of emotional issues, such as depression and anxiety.

Getting your daily omega-6 content from nuts is a healthy option, but you should be aware of it as you choose which foods — and how much of those foods — to eat on a regular basis. For instance, a handful of walnuts is high in both omega-6 and omega-3 fatty acids, making them a wonderful nut choice.

On the Paleo Diet, many of the foods that are rich in omega-6 will disappear from your plate, because many of these foods are man-made and processed foods that didn't appear until after the introduction of the modern Western diet.

Here are the healthy fats we love and highly recommend. Choose the organic versions of them:

✔ **Coconut fats:** Coconuts are an excellent source of saturated fat and produce many delicious varieties of fats. You can use coconut oil in different forms, such as

- **Coconut aminos:** This product is from the sap of a coconut tree and has a salty flavor. Coconut aminos are a great substitute for soy sauce.

- **Coconut oil:** Choose unrefined coconut oil, and use it for sautéing, roasting, and baking in place of vegetable oils and shortening.

- **Unsweetened coconut:** Enjoy flakes as a snack, and use shredded coconut to add fat and sweetness to curries, salads, and desserts.

- **Coconut milk:** You can substitute coconut milk for yogurt and cream in recipes — or splash it into coffee instead of half-and-half.

Make sure that you choose a coconut milk that uses guar gum as a stabilizer. Don't use any others. Avoid the coconut milk in the carton, and use the variety in cans.

✔ **Olives and avocados:** Both olives and avocados are favored sources of monounsaturated fats. Use olive oil and avocado oil for drizzling on salads, and nibble on both olives and avocados in salads or as snacks for healthy fat intake.

Look for packaged olives that contain only water, olives, and salt; avoid chemical additives and stabilizers. Toss them into salads and cooked foods to add healthy fat.

Use only extra-virgin olive oil on salads or drizzle over cooked vegetables and meats. This particular oil has what is known as a *low smoke point,* which means when you add heat, it goes *rancid* (spoils) very quickly. When you eat rancid oil, you run the risk of taking what was once a healthy oil, and making it unhealthy. Unhealthy, rancid oils create inflammation in the body.

✔ **Animal fats:** Animal fats are an excellent choice for cooking, but only if the fats come from organic, grass-fed, pastured animals. If you can find a good source, then fats like lard, tallow, and *ghee* (clarified butter) are healthful, delicious options.

✔ **Nuts, nut oils, and nut butters:** In moderation, nuts and nut butters are tasty options to add fat to meals, snacks, and desserts. Raw or dry roasted are your best bet. Eat them in moderation; add to cooked foods for crunch, or enjoy a few as a snack.

Nut oils are a nice way to add unexpected flavors to salads, but don't use them for cooking, because they become unstable and rancid with heat. For nut butters, examine the label for added sugar. Enjoy nut butters in moderation; they're great for snacks, sauces, and desserts.

Nuts are calorically dense, and you can easily eat a lot of them without realizing just how much you ate. Typically, a single serving of nuts is a quarter cup or about a small handful.

✔ **Seeds:** Seeds are good Paleo-friendly snacks. Some seed choices are pumpkin, sesame, sunflower, and pine nuts.

Don't skimp when budgeting your money on oils, because the right fats and oils can make your cells incredibly healthy, and the opposite is also true. Unhealthy or rancid oils can make you incredibly unhealthy because they create inflammation, whereas healthy oils help inflammation leave the body. Because inflammation is the catalyst for so many problems, adding some healthy fats to your diet can really make a big difference.

On the other hand, some oils are just bad for you. The following oils may get billed as healthy oils, but these industrial and seed oils are very processed and prone to turning rancid, creating inflammation in the body, so stay clear of them as much as possible. They include the following:

- Canola oil
- Corn oil
- Cottonseed oil
- Margarine
- Palm kernel oil
- Partially hydrogenated oil
- Peanut oil
- Safflower oil
- Soybean oil
- Sunflower oil
- Trans fats
- Vegetable shortening

Healthy pantry items

Finding pantry items in-line with your tasting lifestyle can get a little dicey because you have to enter the middle-aisle territory of your grocery store. (When searching for healthy proteins and produce, you can stick to the old nutritional tenet of "stay out of the center aisles and stick to the perimeter of the store.")

The following list eases your shopping anxiety. Everything on this list is nutritious and delicious. Using these flavor enhancers can give your foods great flavor without any added junk. Furthermore, all are gluten free, grain free, dairy free, soy free, legume free, and processed free (just not free; you do have to buy them).

- **Arrowroot powder:** Substitute for flour and cornstarch to thicken soups, stews, and sauces.

- ✔ **Pickles:** Examine labels for added sugar and chemical ingredients, and then enjoy pickles whenever you want a tart bite.

- ✔ **Broth/stock:** Review labels for soy and hidden sugars; use in place of water or wine in sauces, soups, stews, and sautés.

- ✔ **Tomato paste:** Use to add depth of flavor to sauces, soups, and stews.

- ✔ **Canned tomatoes:** Make your own quick marinara sauce or add to soups and stews for a savory touch and extra veggies.

- ✔ **Curry paste:** Examine labels for soy and added sugar. These pastes are great to have on hand to make a quick meal with coconut milk, protein, and veggies.

- ✔ **Canned chiles:** Mild green, jalapeño, or chipotle chile peppers add zing to everyday ingredients. Examine labels for preservatives.

- ✔ **Jarred salsas:** Salsas are great for adding flavor. Examine labels for chemical preservatives, sugar, corn, and wheat.

Avoiding Certain Foods

When you're fasting, not only what you do, but what you don't do can have a major impact. These sections list the foods that you should avoid because they don't bring nutrition to your body; in fact they take away nutrition.

The only way to get lean, strong, and healthy is to bring nutrition into the cells and remove the toxins, which these foods don't do. They actually cause blood sugar disturbances, damage the gut, and cause inflammation in the body, all of which are the precursor to all modern day diseases, premature aging, and weight gain.

In addition to the foods in these sections, you also want to avoid processed or denatured carbohydrates. For instance, think of those crinkly packages that are grab-and-go snacks or 100-calorie packs made with added sugar or sugar substitutes that serve to foolishly lure you into thinking they will help you lose weight. We only approve of carbohydrates from real foods.

Frankenfoods: It's alive!

Frankenfoods are processed soy and meat alternatives made to look like real foods, but they're nothing more than fake foods from head to toe. Think of Dr. Frankenstein making his monster. The same correlates to these food items. Scientists made these freakish foods.

They're and the worst of the worst of processed foods. These foods are genetically engineered, and full of allergens, preservatives, additives, and flavor enhancers.

Unlike soy foods such as edamame, tempeh, and traditional miso, which are closer to their natural state, frankenfoods are a far cry from anything real.

These frankenfoods include

- Tofu hot dogs and burgers
- Veggie loafs
- Veggie sausage links
- Veggie chicken
- Veggie chicken wings
- Veggie bacon

We understand that some vegetarians don't eat any eggs or fish and want to expand their protein sources, which is smart, but we urge people to get their protein elsewhere. These items aren't healthy for anyone. Period. In fact, they aren't even foods; they're food products. They're usually a mixture of a wheat protein with a subpar oil.

If you eat fish, we suggest you try a salmon burger as a healthy swap. They're full of protein and good fats, and a great alternative to some of these frankenfoods, especially for picnics. If you don't eat fish, then we suggest you get your protein from edamame, beans, natto, hemp, tempeh, and tofu.

Understanding sugar

Sugar is sugar is sugar. Some sugars, in moderation, have some slight value, but you should avoid some of them at all costs. The rules for sugar are steadfast throughout any fasting regimen or throughout any healthy diet or weight-loss plan.

Sugar is not only highly addictive (the more you eat the more you crave), but it's also an immunity suppressor. As little as 3.5 ounces can suppress your immune system up to 50 percent. The *American Journal of Clinical Nutrition* published research as early as 1973 that showed that these effects start within an hour of consuming sugar and can last up to five hours.

Most sugar is void of nutrients. In fact, what's really interesting is that it requires nutrients to metabolize sugar, thus pulling minerals from your body. So sugar actually depletes your body of vitamins and minerals. Sugar addiction leads you wide open to every disease from the common cold to cancer. Sugar also impairs your blood cells from doing their job, which is to scavenge bacteria that can make you sick.

We highly recommend that you be pretty picky when you open the sugar gate. This list guides you to the sugars that are okay in moderation, and those that are on the no list. Sugars that are okay in moderation include the following:

- ✔ Coconut (palm) sugar
- ✔ Dates/date sugar
- ✔ Green leaf stevia
- ✔ Fruit juice
- ✔ Maple syrup (organic/grade B)
- ✔ Molasses
- ✔ Raw honey
- ✔ Smashed bananas for baking

Meanwhile, for optimal health and weight loss, you need to eliminate or at the very least moderate all foods with added sugars from your diet, especially those foods with 5 to 10 grams or more of sugar. Four grams of sugar is one teaspoon. Steer clear of these added sugars:

- ✔ Agave
- ✔ Brown sugar
- ✔ Raw sugar
- ✔ Sugar cane
- ✔ White sugar
- ✔ Brown rice sugar
- ✔ Corn syrup
- ✔ High-fructose corn syrup
- ✔ All other packaged, boxed, or packets of highly toxic artificial sugars such as aspartame (NutraSweet or Equal), sucralose (Splenda), processed stevia (Truvia or Sun Crystals), and saccharin.

We understand that avoiding sugar altogether is impossible. Carbohydrates in healthy vegetables and fruits are essentially sugars, and your body runs off of them, so naturally these sugars aren't inherently bad. However, you want to steer clear of artificial sugars because they're toxic to the nervous system and really to your entire body. Don't even bother with them.

Getting the lowdown on salt

Your body needs salt. However, you want to make sure you're consuming the right type of salt. You want to do without *processed* salt — the run-of-the-mill table salt — that is a heavily refined food. Table salt is chemically cleaned with bleach and then mixed with toxic anti-caking agents to make sure the salt flows properly.

Adding the right kind of salt, in the form of sea salt, to your diet during your fasting eating period is important when reducing caloric intake because every structure and function of the body needs minerals to function properly. Your cells need minerals to do their job, and if you reduce calories, you can't do so without making sure you're fulfilling your body's requirement for getting vitamins, minerals, and antioxidants. Sea salts are loaded with trace minerals, including *magnesium* and *potassium*. These two minerals allow fluids to flow in and out of your cells, letting your cell walls become permeable. When your cells are *permeable*, your body naturally releases what it doesn't need. You don't have fluid retention that causes the high blood pressure you hear about with salt intake.

We love Fine Ground Vital Mineral Blend of Celtic Salt (www.celtic-seasalt.com), which is rich in minerals and has no additives. It's very pure and delicious.

Iodine in salt actually isn't natural. Therefore, when you buy unprocessed salt, you won't find iodine in the product. Because you need iodine for your thyroid, hormones, and immune function, make sure you get iodine from other sources, such as the following:

- ✔ Seaweed: Kelp and dulse
- ✔ Protein: Eggs, meat, and poultry
- ✔ Vegetables: Swiss chard, asparagus, and spinach
- ✔ Strawberries

A great way to get iodine is from a delicious product called Sea Snax (http://store.seasnax.com). You can eat these roasted seaweed sheets (which come in large or small) that are naturally rich in iodine as a snack just by themselves or crumble them up in soups or salads.

Watching the booze: Happy hour or not?

During your actual fasting (or non-eating time), you obviously won't be drinking any alcohol. When you're fasting, you're consuming limited calories, so using them on something like alcohol that is void of nutrients wouldn't be a smart choice to fulfill your needs. During your eating window, consuming alcohol isn't the best choice either because you want your liver to process real toxins to keep you healthy and well, instead of processing the alcohol that you drink.

However, we're realists, and we can't negate the positive effects moderate amounts of alcohol can have to help you relax. If you do decide to drink, make wise choices because alcohol is a carcinogen and is toxic to the liver (not to mention its addictive qualities), and go easy.

If you're going to pop a cork, some choices are better than others. Here are our suggestions:

- ✔ Certain types of beer (gluten-free is best)
- ✔ Bourbon
- ✔ Grain-based vodka
- ✔ Gin (some brands are processed with grain-based alcohol)
- ✔ Whisky

For special occasions, consider these options:

- ✔ Tequila
- ✔ Potato vodka
- ✔ Organic red wine
- ✔ Organic sparkling wine
- ✔ Organic white wine

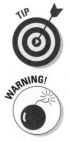

The drier the wine, the less sugar content it has. Try pinot noir, cabernet sauvignon, and merlot for the red wines and sauvignon blanc and Albariño for the whites.

When choosing to celebrate, steer clear of grain-based drinks that can also include gluten, such as beer or rum. These spirits are off-limits 100 percent of the time.

An approved margarita: Add the salt, please

Robb Wolf, biochemist and author of the *New York Times* bestseller *The Paleo Solution* has created a drink that is lower in sugar and better then a lot of choices out there. So if you're going to choose a mixed drink, this is the Infamous NorCal Margarita that we recommend. Just add these three ingredients and enjoy:

- ✔ Two shots of tequila
- ✔ Juice of one lime (yes, an entire lime)
- ✔ A splash of soda water

 Mix spirits with soda water, ice, and a squeeze of fresh lemon or lime juice. Avoid sodas, juices, or tonic water, all which are very high in sugar. Also, when you indulge, get plenty of fat and protein in your belly like maybe a handful of nuts, coconut chips, or avocado wrapped in gluten-free, sulfite-free deli meat.

Making Healthy Cooking Choices

Most people are familiar with good-tasting food because of the more traditional methods of cooking, such as frying, breading, or adding sugary carbohydrates and grains, as well as other additives, to flavor foods. These methods and ingredients aren't going to get you lean, strong, and filled with life and energy.

Because you're invested in living a healthier lifestyle by fasting, and want to look and feel your best, you should take it one step further and discover the cooking methods that give you wellness, not just during your fast, but also forever.

These sections give you the skinny on the best cooking equipment to make your life easier and the preferred cooking methods to live lean, long, and strong.

Easing your life with kitchen essentials

Imagine if you walked into a kitchen and had to stock it from scratch. What equipment would you use if you were on a budget? These cooking tools are the bare-bone essentials for creating awesome recipes with ease. Make your life easy (especially when dealing with a fasting regimen) by having this must-have equipment on the ready.

✔ **Baking sheets:** You should have two large baking sheets with rims, which are ideal for roasting, baking, and catching drips when placed under other pans in the oven.

✔ **Chef's knife:** The chef's knife is the most essential tool of all. The key to a good knife is one that you feel comfortable holding in your hand. A 6- to 10-inch chef's knife is usually the best fit for most, with the 8-inch knife being a popular size. If your budget allows, you may want to look for a high-quality stainless steel knife because you'll be using it so much.

✔ **Sharpening stone:** Cutting produces friction, and this friction causes a knife's blade to go dull, so having a chef's sharpening stone is essential. To sharpen, slide the blade forward and across the stone with moderate pressure, keeping the blade against the stone at an angle. Repeat about ten times.

✔ **Cutting board or mat:** A large wooden cutting board is worth its weight in gold in your kitchen. Wooden cutting boards keep your knives sharp.

You may also want a small plastic board or a cutting mat that's easy to pick up so you can transport the food easily wherever you want it. Plastic boards are great for trimming meats and are easy to clean up.

✔ **Colander:** A colander is a must for draining fatty meats or steamed vegetables and for washing produce.

✔ **Food processor or blender:** When you start preparing healthy foods, you'll find these appliances irreplaceable. Technically, you don't need both. Although having both is nice, you can definitely get away with one or the other. Some people have a preference for a food processor while others prefer to use the blender. These tools are great for creating fantastic sauces and soups. The food processor also makes slicing vegetables fast and easy.

✔ **Food storage containers:** Your best bet to keep your kitchen immune-boosting is to use containers that are fee of the toxin BPA, found in plastics. Instead, opt for stackable glass containers with tight-sealing lids. These containers work well for transporting and freezing food, too.

✔ **Food thermometer:** Using an instant-read thermometer is a safeguard everyone should take. When you're cooking meat, knowing the internal temperature is crucial.

✔ **Measuring cups and spoons:** Measuring cups that range in size from a quarter cup to 1 cup and measuring spoons from a quarter teaspoon to 1 tablespoon satisfy the needs for any cooking rendezvous. You may want two sets so you don't always have to wash them while you're cooking.

✔ **Mixing bowls:** Durable mixing bowls in a range of sizes are always handy for prep work and tossing.

✔ **Paring knife:** For smaller tasks, like slicing an apple or peeling something, the paring knife is your go-to tool. Again, use one that feels good in your hand.

✔ **Pots and pans:** A few simple pans can make your life easier.

- **Large, deep baking pan:** They're great for roasting vegetables and making casseroles.

- **Large sauté pan:** They're perfect for sautés and stir-fries. A 12-inch pan ought to do it.

- **Large soup pot:** You'll wonder how you survived without this pot. Get one larger than you think you need.

- **Large wok:** This piece is handy for when you want a quick, throw-together meal.

✔ **Small and large saucepans:** You'll use these pans for a number of dishes.

These pots and pans shouldn't be nonstick. They should be ceramic, glass, or stainless steel, preferably made in the United States or Europe, to avoid toxins used in nonstick materials.

Recognizing cooking methods

You certainly don't have to be a gourmet chef to use healthy cooking techniques. Anyone can use these simple methods to prepare foods that lock in high-octane flavor and provide deep nutrition. Here we explain some favorite eating-window cooking methods that are simple and still preserve the natural nutrition in your foods. No matter whether you're in your fasting mindset or not, you should apply these healthy cooking practices whenever you step in the kitchen.

No matter what method you use to cook your food, using spices and herbs is one of the best ways to add color, flavor, and aroma to your meals. Choose fresh herbs that are bright and have a pungent color and aren't wilted. Always add them toward the end of cooking. If you're using dried herbs, you can add them to the earlier stages of cooking. Go ahead and experiment and use as many spices as you can get you hands on.

Baking

You don't have to add anything extra to food when you bake. You place lean meats, seafood, poultry, vegetables, or even fruit in a pan or dish either uncovered or covered. The hot, dry air of your oven turns these foods into something special — without the extra calories or fat. Try baking some of the denser carbohydrates, such as squash or sweet potatoes. The heat caramelizes the natural sugars, making for a delicious side dish.

Braising

Braising is a fantastic method to use for inexpensive, tougher cuts of meat, because you can turn them into tender meats just by using this easy cooking method. When braising meats, first brown them on high heat to caramelize the outside, and then slowly cook them in flavored liquid, like water or broth, to make the meat tender and lock in all its flavors. You can even use this liquid afterward for a flavorful, nutrient-rich sauce. You can braise meat in a covered pan in the oven or on the stove top in a heavy pot with a tight-fitting lid. You can simmer the meat in water, or you can add herbs, spices, and vegetables.

Sautéing and stir-frying

Sautéing and stir-frying are similar cooking methods and great for adding flavor to thinly sliced, uniformly sized meat and vegetables. With just a little fat and a skillet, you pan-cook meat and vegetables until they're browned. When the ingredients brown, this means they've caramelized, adding a burst of natural flavors to your dish. Simply by adding olive oil, some of your favorite seasonings, and herbs tossed in at the end, you can create a hearty, unbelievably tasty dish.

Roasting

Roasting is the perfect no-frills, super-nutritious way to prepare a meal for your family in a snap. Three words describe roasting: *Simple, healthy,* and *delicious.* Place chicken or beef roast in a pan, surround it with hearty vegetables, and put it in the oven for a few hours. The meat cooks in its natural juices, and you can simmer and strain the drippings in the bottom of the pan to create a sauce.

Slow cooking

Slow cooking may be the most perfect way of cooking on the planet. If you're busy and enjoy warm, hearty meals, you'll love the magic of the slow cooker. You can make just about anything you can think of in a slow cooker while you're running around with kids, at work, or just relaxing. Meats and vegetables cook on low temperatures over longer periods of time than other cooking methods, so the meat gets tender and the flavors blend together, creating that slow cook magic.

Steaming

Steaming is as basic at it gets and is how you really get the nutrition locked in your vegetables. The steam holds the nutrients in the vegetables, brightening their color and making them inviting to eat. You can even flavor the liquid by adding seasonings to the water, which brings out even more flavor as they cook.

Poaching

To poach foods, slowly simmer ingredients in either water or a broth until they're cooked thoroughly and are tender. The food retains its shape and texture with the benefit of not drying out, leaving it tender and delicious. Poaching is a great way to cook fish so it's tender and flavorful.

Batch cooking

If you want to stay on board with your fasting foods, batch cooking is the way to go. Batch cooking helps you organize your time so you always have healthy food and family staples on hand. It also saves you time and money because you always know exactly what you need at the grocery store, which means you make fewer trips and buy less food that you don't use or need.

Here's how it works: You devote one or two days a week to spending an hour or so in the kitchen preparing foods that your family eats on a regular basis. Precook as many staple or convenience foods as you can. Prepare foods like hard-boiled eggs, cut and chop veggies, precook meats, make salads, and prepare dips or sauces, such as guacamole. Stick the food in storage containers, label them, put them in the fridge or freezer, and you have your own personal restaurant for the week.

Schedule your batching days as a routine part of your week. When you do, cooking becomes so much less of a chore — it may even be fun. After a couple of times, you get super quick, and it becomes no big deal.

The more access you have to real foods, the better you'll feel and the more you'll get done regardless of time crunches. You can organize your way into more time and a healthier immune-boosting life.

Grilling — Limit the amount you use it

Grilling cooks food over direct heat on a grill rack above a bed of charcoal or gas-heated rocks. Although grilling is certainly a warm-weather favorite and the center of many fun gatherings, go easy on grilling and don't make it your everyday cooking method.

Here's why: When you grill food, proteins are damaged and carcinogens are produced. Evidence shows that *heterocyclic amines* (HCAs) produced in meat when cooked at high temperature are carcinogenic. This risk is increased when the meat is cooked well done. When you add refined oils in marinades and directly on the grill, you can suppress the immune system and increase the risks for cancer.

You can take action to minimize your exposure by using the following tips:

- **Don't use grilling as your go-to cooking method:** Incorporate other cooking methods mentioned in this section to your cooking repertoire.

- **Ditch the processed vegetable oils:** On marinades or directly on the grill, opt for saturated fats, which can withstand high heat without becoming rancid. Coconut oil and grass-fed butter are great options. (See the section "Healthy fats," earlier in this chapter.)

- **Veggie up:** When you eat grilled foods, pile on the vegetables. The phenols and antioxidants (*phenols* are healing properties from plants and *antioxidants* are nutrients that protect the body and can prevent cancers) in them soften the impact of the mutations caused by the grilled meats.

- **Don't overheat:** Keep meat away from direct heat or let juices fall on the heat source. Make sure you don't overcook or char the food, which greatly increases the carcinogens.

Chapter 9

For Women: 500-Calorie Meal Recipes

In This Chapter

▶ Discovering non-inflammatory recipes

▶ Adding variety on your 5:2 Diet days with these easy, delicious 250-calorie per serving meals

*E*ating only 500-calories a day has always been easy — if you starved yourself. Imagine those limited-calorie frozen dinners, each with under 300 calories. The portions are so tiny that they seem more like appetizers than entrees. And they're often full of cheap ingredients you would never cook yourself.

The good news is that you can limit your calorie intake to 500 calories, and you don't have to starve, and you can eat real food and be satisfied. The trick is to fill up on protein, healthy fat, and fiber, and limit calorie-bomb simple carbohydrates, such as white flour and sugar. Protein can come from animal or vegetable sources, and fiber from vegetables and fruits.

Cooking will not only teach you about portion control and quality ingredients, but you can also eat real food if you cook it yourself.

The recipes in this chapter are each about 500 calorie or about 250 calories per portion (A few recipes have slightly more than 250 calories per serving. You'll just need to adjust accordingly your food intake for the day to stay under 500 calories.). They're easy to prepare with simple ingredients that are grain-free and dairy-free. By eating these protein-rich meals (which keep you satisfied for a long time after you eat them), and adding bulk in the form of vegetables, healthy fats, and fruits, you actually can have your lunch and dinner, and eat them too.

You can mix and match these meals as much as you want. Even better, most of these recipes feed two people, so you can either make enough for yourself for two meals or share with another person. You can also double or triple the recipes to feed a crowd.

Head to www.dummies.com/extras/fastdiets for a few more 500-calorie recipes.

Going the Beef Route

You may think that 500 calories can be quite a lot of food, but it only is if you're eating only vegetables. By adding protein-rich foods, such as lean beef, trimmed of as much fat as possible, you're actually going to feel more satisfied for a longer time after eating. Eating smaller portions of high-quality protein allows you to eat less food because lean protein is slower to digest in the body — so that by the time your body digests the beef, it's likely time to eat again.

Of course, the key to eating any meat is the word *lean*. That's why you purchase beef (as well as poultry, fish, and other meats) from reputable sources.

These recipes utilize many different cuts of beef as their main ingredient. The beef is always trimmed of as much as possible of visible fat and paired with bulky vegetables and seasoning that turns a sometimes-boring meal into a complete dining experience. We also include dishes with international flavors, which can help keep cooking and eating interesting and satisfying.

Recipes in This Chapter (contd.)

- ► Seared Scallops with Tomato Basil Salad
- ► Broiled Tilapia with Cucumber Salsa
- ► Shrimp and Kelp Noodle Salad
- ► Basil and Bell Pepper Shrimp Kebabs
- ► Quick Pork and Vegetable Stir Fry
- ► Egg White Prosciutto and Vegetable Frittata
- ► Greek Lamb Tacos
- ► Spinach Salad with Carrots, Tomatoes, Blueberries, and Honey Mustard Vinaigrette
- ► Dijon Egg White Salad
- ► Roasted Vegetable Lettuce Sandwiches
- ► "Spaghetti" with Eggplant Ragu
- ► Fresh Fruit Salad with Coconut Cream

Skinny Slow-Cooked Chili

Prep time: 30 min • **Cook time:** 5 hr • **Yield:** 2 servings

Ingredients	Directions
8 ounces very lean ground beef	**1** In a large nonstick skillet, brown the ground beef over medium-high heat, stirring often to break up lumps.
1 cup water	
1 cup canned diced tomatoes with juice	**2** Place the browned beef in a small (3- to 4-quart) slow cooker with all the ingredients except the zucchini. Cover and cook 4 hours on the low setting. Add the zucchini, stir well, and cook for another hour.
¼ cup chopped celery	
¼ chopped onions	
2 teaspoons medium chili powder	**3** Season with salt and pepper to taste, and serve hot, garnished with the scallions.
2½ teaspoons minced garlic	
Pinch red pepper flakes or more	
Pinch dried oregano	
½ teaspoon fine sea salt	
Fresh ground black pepper	
1 cup quarter-inch diced zucchini	
2 tablespoons chopped scallions	

Per serving: Calories 192; Total fat: 6g; Saturated fat: 2g; Cholesterol: 60mg; Sodium: 1,067mg; Carbohydrates: 14g; Fiber: 3g; Sugar: 6g; Protein: 25g.

Tip: The beef must be very lean for this, recipe to be calorie friendly. Use at least 95 percent lean beef. You can also substitute white-meat chicken or turkey breast for the beef.

(Recipe by Annabel Cohen)

Seared Beef Tenderloin with Mushrooms and Cauliflower with Truffle Salt

Prep time: 20 min • **Cook time:** 15 min • **Yield:** 2 servings

Ingredients	Directions
4 cups cauliflower florets	*1* Place the cauliflower in a microwave-safe bowl with ¼ cup of water and cover with plastic wrap. Cook on high power for 6 to 8 minutes, until tender (check after 6 minutes). Use a fork to smash the cauliflower, and season with truffle salt and place back in the microwave oven.
¼ cup water	
Truffle salt to taste	
8 ounces center-cut beef tenderloin	
8 ounces sliced mushrooms	*2* Spray a large nonstick skillet with nonstick cooking spray and heat over medium-high heat. Add the beef to the pan and cook for 5 to 6 minutes (for medium-rare) on all sides or until the desired degree of doneness. Remove to a plate and set aside. Add the mushrooms to the pan, add a bit of salt and pepper and thyme, and sauté until the mushrooms just give up their liquid. Lightly season with more salt and pepper if desired.
½ teaspoon fine sea salt	
1 teaspoon fresh thyme or ¼ teaspoon dried	
¼ teaspoon fresh ground pepper	
	3 Heat the cauliflower until hot or warm by cooking in the microwave on high for about 2 minutes.
	4 Slice the beef against the grain into half-inch slices. Serve the beef with the cauliflower and mushrooms. Drizzle the collected juices from the beef and mushrooms over the top.

Per serving: Calories 248; Total fat: 8g; Saturated fat: 3g; Cholesterol: 67mg; Sodium: 974mg; Carbohydrates: 15g; Fiber: 7g; Sugar: 6g; Protein: 32 g.

(Recipe by Annabel Cohen)

Focus on non-inflammatory foods and stop your leaky gut

If you want to look and feel your best, you have to keep the inflammation out of your body, whether you're fasting or not. Inflammation is the precursor to just about every modern-day disease known today, including heart disease, cancer, diabetes, and more. By using good old back-to-nature real foods, you can spare yourself from what is known as *gut-inflammation* or leaky gut.

Here's the story behind leaky gut: Your gut is basically a big tube (25 feet long) where your immune system has to figure out which abnormal bacteria to fight, which bacteria are helpful, and which bacteria to leave alone.

Your gut's lining has to be strong and healthy in order to create a healing wall that doesn't allow anything to penetrate. It has tiny, finger-like projections called *villi*, which is where the absorption of nutrients takes place. If these villi are damaged, then nutrients aren't properly absorbed. Worse yet, this damage can cause some undigested food and bacteria to go through the healing wall and enter the bloodstream where it doesn't belong. If your body doesn't recognize an invader, it will attack itself instead of protecting, which is what it's designed to do. An immune response happens and inflammation occurs, which is when you get autoimmune problems (like diabetes, thyroid problems, arthritic problems, Crohn's disease, and more), chronic disease, unexplained fatigue, intestinal distress, allergies, and hypersensitivities to everything.

The recipes in this chapter include ingredients that are the mainstay foods for creating healing within the body by creating a strong, healthy gut, which can get you well, keep you well, help you look amazing, drop the pounds, and perform your best.

Whipping Up Some Poultry

Like beef, the protein from skinless and boneless chicken breast meat and turkey breast meat is extremely lean. In animal products, protein is located in the muscle tissue. This lean protein digests slowly in the body, leading to feelings of fullness for longer.

White meat, boneless and skinless chicken breast meat, and turkey breast meat boast about 30 calories per ounce, which means you can eat quite a bit of poultry as part of this very low-calorie staple of your fast regime. And because the flavor of poultry is mild, pairs well with so many other ingredients, and cooks quickly, It's easy to prepare in so many different ways.

The following recipes include poultry in fresh salads, exotic stir fries, elegant entrees, roasted choices, and even a big burger. Each is easy to prepare, yet tastes like restaurant-quality meals.

Chinese Chicken Napa Salad

Prep time: 15 min • **Cook time:** None • **Yield:** 2 servings

Ingredients	Directions
6 ounces baked, broiled, or grilled chicken breasts, boneless and skinless	**1** Shred the chicken with your fingers into thin pieces and place in a large bowl. Add the remaining salad ingredients and toss.
4 cups shredded Napa or Chinese cabbage	
1 cup snow peas, thinly sliced	**2** Combine the dressing ingredients in a small bowl and whisk well. Pour the dressing over the salad and toss well. Add salt and pepper to taste and toss again.
1 cup mung bean sprouts	
½ cup shredded or crated carrots	
¼ cup chopped scallions	
1 tablespoon slivered almonds	

Dressing

1 tablespoon honey

2 tablespoons coconut aminos

2 tablespoons red-wine vinegar

1 tablespoon olive oil

Salt and pepper to taste

Per serving: Calories 295; Total fat: 11g; Saturated fat: 2g; Cholesterol: 47mg; Sodium: 718mg; Carbohydrates: 28g; Fiber: 6g; Sugar: 16g; Protein: 23g.

Note: Mung bean sprouts are beans that are just sprouting, are about 2–3 inches long, and often are used in Asian cooking. You can find them in most supermarkets and Asian food stores.

(Recipe by Annabel Cohen)

Chicken Cobb Salad

Prep time: 15 min • **Cook time:** None • **Yield:** 2 servings

Ingredients	Directions
5 cups chopped Romaine lettuce	**1** Arrange the lettuce on two dinner-size plates.
6 ounces chopped cooked, boneless, and skinless chicken breasts (baked or grilled)	**2** Top the lettuce with chicken, arranged in a strip. Next to the chicken, arrange the tomatoes, eggs, cucumber, beets, and carrots in individual strips over the lettuce.
½ cup chopped plum tomatoes	**3** Combine the dressing ingredients in a medium bowl and whisk well. Drizzle the dressing over the salad and serve.
4 eggs, hard-boiled, white parts only, chopped	
1 cup diced cucumber, unpeeled	
½ cup diced, cooked beets	
½ cup shredded carrots	

Dressing

3 tablespoons red-wine vinegar

½ tablespoon cold-pressed olive oil

1 tablespoon Dijon mustard

Fine sea salt and fresh ground pepper to taste

Per serving: Calories 284; Total fat: 11g; Saturated fat: 2g; Cholesterol: 72mg; Sodium: 701mg; Carbohydrates: 15g; Fiber: 5g; Sugar: 8g; Protein: 37g.

Vary It: You don't have to make this as a Cobb salad with all ingredients separated. Feel free to toss this salad instead.

(Recipe by Annabel Cohen)

Chopped Chicken and Roasted Pear Salad with Honey Vinaigrette

Prep time: 15 min • **Cook time:** 15 min • **Yield:** 2 servings

Ingredients	Directions
1 ripe pear (any variety), unpeeled, quartered lengthwise, cored and cut into 1-inch cubes	**1** Preheat the oven to 400°F. Line a baking sheet with parchment.
1 teaspoon cold-pressed extra-virgin olive oil	**2** Toss the pear cubes with the olive oil in a medium bowl, and arrange the pear cubes on the prepared baking sheet. Roast for 12 minutes. Remove from the oven and cool.
6 ounces cooked, boneless, and skinless chicken breasts, chopped	
4 cups mixed baby or field greens	**3** To make the dressing, whisk together the dressing ingredients in a small bowl and set aside.
1 cup seedless cucumber	**4** Combine the pear, chicken, mixed greens, and cucumber in a large bowl. Drizzle the dressing on the salad, toss gently, and serve.
Fine sea salt and fresh ground pepper, to taste	

Dressing

2 teaspoons cold-pressed extra-virgin olive oil

2 teaspoons honey

2 tablespoons fresh lemon juice

Per serving: Calories 248; Total fat: 10g; Saturated fat: 2g; Cholesterol: 72mg; Sodium: 425mg; Carbohydrates: 13g; Fiber: 2g; Sugar: 7g; Protein: 29 g.

Vary It: Change the pear to apple if desired and add ½-cup additional chopped fresh herbs to vary this salad to your own tastes.

(Recipe by Annabel Cohen)

Chicken Caesar Salad with Almonds

Prep time: 15 min • **Cook time:** 10 min • **Yield:** 2 servings

Ingredients	*Directions*
1 boneless and skinless chicken breast (about 6 ounces), trimmed of all fat	*1* Heat a large nonstick skillet over medium-high heat. Spray with nonstick cooking spray. Add the chicken to the pan, and cook 4 to 5 minutes on each side or until just cooked through (don't overcook).
2 tablespoons sliced or slivered almonds	
6 cups chopped Romaine lettuce	*2* Remove the chicken to a cutting board to cool for 5 minutes. Cut against the grain into half-inch slices.
Celtic sea salt and fresh ground pepper to taste	*3* Combine the dressing ingredients in a small bowl and whisk well to mash the anchovies.
	4 Place the lettuce and almonds in a large bowl. Add the dressing and chicken and toss well. Serve with fresh ground pepper to taste.

Dressing

2 anchovies packed in oil, drained (optional)

1 tablespoon red-wine vinegar

1 tablespoon fresh lemon juice

1 tablespoon olive oil

½ teaspoon minced garlic or more to taste

1 teaspoon Dijon mustard

Per serving: Calories 213; Total fat: 12g; Saturated fat: 2g; Cholesterol: 47mg; Sodium: 353mg; Carbohydrates: 7g; Fiber: 4g; Sugar: 2g; Protein: 20g.

(Recipe by Annabel Cohen)

Turkey Salad with Grapefruit, Almonds, and Curried Coconut Dressing

Prep time: 5 min • **Cook time:** None • **Yield:** 2 servings

Ingredients	Directions
8 ounces cooked turkey breast meat, cut into 1-inch chunks	**1** Combine all the ingredients in a large bowl and toss well to coat. Season with salt and pepper to taste.
1 medium grapefruit, peeled, divided into sections, and cut into 1-inch chunks	
¾ cup chopped celery	
¼ cup slivered almonds	
2 tablespoons cilantro leaves, chopped	
¼ cup coconut cream	
2 tablespoons fresh lemon juice	
1 teaspoon curry powder	
½ teaspoon minced garlic	
Fine sea salt and fresh ground pepper to taste	

Per serving: Calories 404; Total fat: 18g; Saturated fat: 10g; Cholesterol: 94mg; Sodium: 382mg; Carbohydrates: 23g; Fiber: 5g; Sugar: 13g; Protein: 40g.

Vary It: Change the spices, herbs, fruits, and nuts to your own tastes.

Note: Delete the almonds to make this recipe about 300 calories per serving.

(Recipe by Annabel Cohen)

Lemon, Wine, and Basil-Sautéed Chicken with Spinach and Mushrooms

Prep time: 15 min • **Cook time:** 10 min • **Yield:** 2 servings

Ingredients	Directions
½ cup chopped onions	**1** Heat the oil in a large nonstick skillet over medium heat. Add the onions and garlic and sauté for one minute.
½ teaspoon minced garlic	
1 boneless and skinless chicken breast, about 8 ounces	**2** Add the chicken and cook for 2 minutes. Turn the chicken over and cook for one more minute. Lightly season with salt and pepper.
Fine sea salt and fresh ground pepper to taste	
½ cup dry white wine	**3** Add the wine and lemon juice and bring to a boil.
2 tablespoons fresh lemon juice	**4** Add the mushrooms and cook for one minute more. Add the spinach and basil and cover the skillet with a lid. Cook for 2 more minutes. Remove the skillet from the stove, but keep the lid on for another 3 minutes.
¼ cup fresh basil	
8 ounces sliced mushrooms, any variety	
6 cups fresh baby spinach	
	5 To serve, arrange the vegetables on two plates and arrange the chicken over them. Drizzle the pan juices over the dish.

Per serving: Calories 205; Total fat: 3g; Saturated fat: 1g; Cholesterol: 63mg; Sodium: 483mg; Carbohydrates: 17g; Fiber: 6g; Sugar: 4g; Protein: 29g.

Tip: If you're using a large chicken breast instead of two smaller breast halves, butterfly the chicken by cutting it in half, horizontally, into two thinner breast halves.

Vary It: You can substitute asparagus or broccoli for the mushroom.

(Recipe by Annabel Cohen)

Baked Chicken and Salsa Stuffed–Sweet Potatoes

Prep time: 15 min • **Cook time:** 45 min • **Yield:** 2 servings

Ingredients	Directions
2 medium (about 6 ounces each) sweet potatoes	*1* Preheat the oven to 400°F.
4 ounces chopped cooked chicken breasts **¼ cup coconut cream**	*2* Wash the sweet potatoes and prick several times with a fork. Place them on a baking sheet and cook for about 30 to 40 minutes, until a knife inserted in the potato comes out clean. Alternately, microwave the potato on high heat for about 5 minutes. Check to ensure the potato is tender, or cook in 2-minute intervals until tender.
	3 While the potatoes are cooking, combine the salsa ingredients in a small bowl and mix well. Add salt and pepper to taste. Cut large slit lengthwise in the potatoes and carefully press the ends of the potatoes toward the center to open up the slits. Spoon the chicken over the potatoes and top with the salsa and the coconut cream.

Salsa

1 cup chopped Roma or plum tomatoes

1 cup chopped cucumbers, unpeeled

2 tablespoons chopped cilantro

2 tablespoons fresh lemon juice

Salt and pepper to taste

Per serving: Calories 255; Total fat: 10g; Saturated fat: 10g; Cholesterol: 48mg; Sodium: 381mg; Carbohydrates: 35g; Fiber: 6g; Sugar: 12g; Protein: 22g.

(Recipe by Annabel Cohen)

Big Turkey Vegetable Burgers

Prep time: 10 min • **Cook time:** 8 min • **Yield:** 2 servings

Ingredients	Directions
10 ounces extra-lean ground turkey, white meat only (90 percent or more lean)	**1** Combine all the turkey patty ingredients in a medium bowl. Mash with your hands to mix well.
1 egg white	**2** Form into 2 burgers. Chill for at least 15 minutes or up to a day ahead until ready to cook.
3 tablespoons shredded carrots	
3 tablespoons shredded zucchini	**3** To cook, brush a large skillet with olive oil. Heat over medium-high heat until hot. Add the burgers and cook on both sides until just cooked through, about 8 minutes, total. Don't overcook.
3 tablespoons chopped onion	
2 tablespoons chopped fresh parsley	
¼ teaspoon ground cumin	**4** Serve between slices of lettuce leaves, topped with tomatoes, cucumbers, and a drizzle of coconut aminos.
¼ teaspoon fine sea salt	
¼ teaspoon hot pepper sauce	
½ teaspoon olive oil, for cooking	
Iceberg lettuce leaves	
2 large tomato slices	
12 cucumber slices	
1 teaspoon coconut aminos (optional)	

Per serving: Calories 231; Total fat: 2g; Saturated fat: 0g; Cholesterol: 117mg; Sodium: 425 mg; Carbohydrates: 5g; Fiber: 1g; Sugar:2 g; Protein: 45g.

Tip: Ketchup adds sugar and calories, so stick with yellow mustard, if desired, on your burger.

(Recipe by Annabel Cohen)

Serving Some Seafood Dishes

Seafood, and fish in general, is an increasingly popular low-calorie food when compared to other protein-rich foods, such as meat and poultry. Many lean fish varieties contain similar calories per ounce as lean poultry, about 30 to 35 calories. Some of the fattier fishes, of which salmon is one, contain about double that number. The key to eating any protein is the word *lean*. That's why you want to make sure you purchase your fish from reputable sources.

Seafood also contains a high-quality protein and amino acids, making it a complete protein source. Lean fish is also low in both total fat and saturated fat — as a general rule, the lighter the fish, the leaner it is.

These recipes include fresh fish, shellfish, and even canned tuna fish. They're used in salads, stir fries, and grilled and roasted combinations, including a couple with a sweet flavor profile that includes honey as an ingredient.

Nourishing your body's cells

Discovering fasting and the foods that work best within your body are important steps to look and feel your best. If fasting seems intimidating, strict, and even hard, remember what's truly hard — healing your body of serious disease or going through the depression of knowing that you're not living your life because you're tired, in pain, or overweight. From this perspective, understanding these fasting and food principles is just a drop in the bucket. At times, it may take some grit, but it's well worth the effort to get from where you are now to where you want to be.

The fluid around your cells is your internal milieu; this fluid must be healthy for you to be healthy. Think of your body like a fish tank. The water in your tank is your internal milieu. When you eat healthy and balanced food, you nourish this milieu. When you eat poorly, you clog and acidify this system, your cells become like sludge, and you look and feel toxic — like fish trying to survive in a dirty tank. Chapter 8 mentions some foods that will clean out your fish tank and give your body a recharge.

Mediterranean Tuna Salad with Fresh Fennel

Prep time: 15 min • **Cook time:** None • **Yield:** 2 servings

Ingredients	Directions
2 cans (about 5–6 ounces each) albacore white tuna, packed in water	*1* Combine all the ingredients in a medium bowl and toss well.
½ cup chopped fennel bulb	
½ cup chopped celery	
½ cup chopped red or yellow pepper	
1 tablespoon fresh dill	
2 teaspoons cold-pressed extra-virgin olive oil	
2 tablespoons fresh lemon juice or more to taste	
2 tablespoons fresh chopped parsley	
Fine sea salt and fresh ground pepper to taste	

Per serving: Calories 246; Total fat: 9g; Saturated fat: 2g; Cholesterol: 59 mg; Sodium: 860mg; Carbohydrates: 5g; Fiber: 2g; Sugar: 2g; Protein: 34g.

Note: Figure 9-1 shows how to chop fennel.

Tip: To make a larger salad, serve over a bed of chopped lettuce, any variety.

(Recipe by Annabel Cohen)

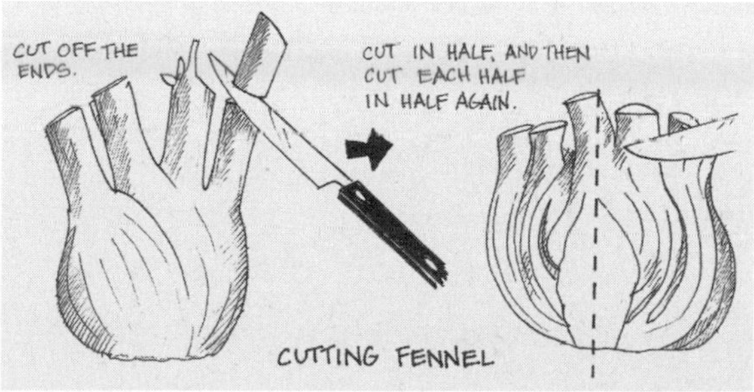

Figure 9-1: How to chop a fennel bulb.

CUT OFF THE ENDS.

CUT IN HALF AND THEN CUT EACH HALF IN HALF AGAIN.

CUTTING FENNEL

Illustrations by Elizabeth Kurtzman

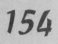

Honey and Lemon Sesame Tuna

Prep time: 15 min • **Cook time:** 4 min • **Yield:** 2 servings

Ingredients	Directions
2 tablespoons coconut aminos	*1* Combine the coconut aminos, fresh lemon juice, and honey in a medium bowl and whisk well.
2 tablespoons fresh lemon juice	
1 teaspoon honey	*2* Add the tuna and turn over several times to coat well. Cover and chill for 30 minutes or more.
One 8-ounce tuna steak	
1 teaspoon coconut oil	*3* Heat the oil in a large skillet over high heat. Add the marinated tuna (discard any remaining marinade). Sear on one side for 2 minutes. Carefully turn the tuna over and sear on the other side for 1 to 2 minutes more, for rare, or a bit more for medium-rare.
Fine sea salt and fresh ground pepper to taste	
1 tablespoon sesame seeds	
2 tablespoons finely chopped scallions	*4* Remove the tuna from the pan and allow the fish to stand for 2 minutes. To serve, slice the tuna into quarter-inch slices and serve with any pan juices drizzled over it. Sprinkle with sesame seeds and scallions.

Per serving: *Calories 229; Total fat: 5g; Saturated fat: 2g; Cholesterol: 53mg; Sodium: 700mg; Carbohydrates: 8g; Fiber: 1g; Sugar: 3g; Protein: 34g.*

Tip: If you remove the honey from the marinade, you can serve the tuna with 1½ cups steamed sugar snap peas if desired.

(Recipe by Annabel Cohen)

Roast Salmon and Asparagus with Honey, Lime, and Cumin

Prep time: 15 min • **Cook time:** 30 min • **Yield:** 2 servings

Ingredients	*Directions*
Two 4-ounce fresh skinless and boneless salmon fillets **8 ounces trimmed asparagus spears** **Fine sea salt and fresh ground pepper to taste**	*1* Preheat the oven to 450°F. Spray a rimmed baking sheet with nonstick cooking spray. Arrange the fish on the baking sheet and season lightly with salt. Arrange the asparagus next to the salmon.
	2 Combine the glaze ingredients in a small bowl and stir well. Drizzle the asparagus with some of the glaze, and then the salmon with the remaining glaze.
	3 Cook the fish and asparagus in the center of the oven for 8 to 10 minutes.
	4 Serve the fish with the asparagus on the side.

Glaze

1 tablespoon honey

2 tablespoons fresh lime juice

1 teaspoon coconut aminos

1 teaspoon grated, peeled fresh gingerroot

¼ teaspoon ground cumin

¼ teaspoon ground cinnamon

Per serving: Calories 211; Total fat: 5g; Saturated fat: 1g; Cholesterol: 53mg; Sodium: 548mg; Carbohydrates: 15g; Fiber: 3g; Sugar: 10g; Protein: 26g.

Tip: Fish and vegetables cook quickly and continue to cook even when you take them out of the oven. This fish cooks in about 8 to 10 minutes per inch of fish thickness. Don't be tempted to overcook the fish or the vegetables.

Tip: Make sure the asparagus is about 5 inches long when trimmed of the tough ends, about 2–3 inches from the bottom. The tough ends are difficult to chew.

(Recipe by Annabel Cohen)

Roast Salmon with Balsamic Vegetables

Prep time: 15 min • **Cook time:** 12 min • **Yield:** 2 servings

Ingredients	Directions
6 ounces salmon, boneless and skinless and cut into two portions	*1* Preheat the oven to 450°F. Spray a rimmed baking dish with nonstick cooking spray. Arrange the salmon portions on the baking sheet. Lightly season with salt and pepper and set aside.
½ teaspoon minced garlic	
1 red bell pepper, cut into thin strips	*2* Place all the remaining ingredients in a large bowl and toss well with your hands. Add salt and pepper to taste and toss well again. Arrange the vegetables around the salmon.
6 ounces thin-sliced mushrooms	
3 ounces pea pods	
3 tablespoons balsamic vinegar	*3* Cook the salmon and vegetables for 7 to 8 minutes, until the salmon is just cooked through. Cool for a minute before serving.
½ teaspoon hot pepper sauce	
1 teaspoon olive oil	

Per serving: Calories 208; Total fat: 6g; Saturated fat: 1g; Cholesterol: 40mg; Sodium: 132mg; Carbohydrates: 14g; Fiber: 3g; Sugar: 9g; Protein: 23g.

Vary It: Alter the fish choices and vegetables in this recipe to make it your own.

Note: Figure 9-2 shows how you can remove pin bones from salmon fillets.

(Recipe by Annabel Cohen)

Figure 9-2: A pair of tweezers helps to remove tiny pin bones from salmon fillets.

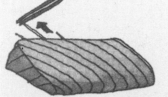

Remove any pin bones in the salmon fillets!

Illustrations by Elizabeth Kurtzman

Foil-Roasted Chili Mahi-Mahi with Avocado and Cabbage

Prep time: 5 min • **Cook time:** 10 min • **Yield:** 2 servings

Ingredients	Instructions
8 ounces boneless mahi-mahi fillets (or your favorite fish) **4 cups shredded Napa or Savoy cabbage** **1 cup chopped ripe tomatoes** **½ medium ripe avocado, sliced** **Fresh lime wedges** **2 tablespoons fresh cilantro, chopped** **½ teaspoon cold-pressed extra virgin olive oil**	**1** Preheat the oven to 400°F. Cut two sheets of heavy-duty aluminum foil about 14-inches long each. Stack the sheets of foil, and spray the top one with nonstick cooking spray. Rinse the fish (but don't dry). Set aside.
	2 Make the rub by combining the salt, pepper, chili powder, cilantro, oregano, and garlic, and rub the mixture over all sides of the fish with your hands.
	3 Place half of the cabbage on each length of foil. Top the cabbage with the fish and add the tomatoes to the fish. Wrap the fish in the foil, sealing the top edge (it should be loose around the cabbage and fish).
	4 Place the fish packets in the oven and cook for 20 minutes (don't overcook). Remove the ingredients of the packets to dinner-size plates. Top with the avocado slices and fresh cilantro and drizzle with the olive oil.

Rub

½ teaspoon fine sea salt

¼ teaspoon fresh ground pepper

2 teaspoons medium chili powder

2 tablespoons fresh chopped cilantro

½ teaspoon dried oregano

¼ teaspoon granulated garlic

Per serving: Calories 245; Total fat: 9g; Saturated fat: 1g; Cholesterol: 80mg; Sodium: 853mg; Carbohydrates: 21g; Fiber: 10g; Sugar: 6g; Protein: 26g.

Note: Cooking in foil is similar to a French cooking technique that calls for cooking in parchment packets called en papillote

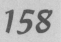

Seared Scallops with Tomato Basil Salad

Prep time: 15 min • **Cook time:** 10 min • **Yield:** 2 servings

Ingredients	Directions
8 ounces large sea scallops	*1* Rinse and dry the scallops well with paper towel. Brush each scallop very lightly with oil. Lightly season with salt and pepper.
1 teaspoon melted coconut oil	
Fine sea salt and fresh ground pepper to taste	*2* Heat a large nonstick skillet over high heat until hot. Add the scallops and cook for 1 minute. Turn the scallops over and cook on the other side, for about 2 minutes for medium-rare (longer if your prefer your scallops well done).
	3 While the scallops are cooking, toss all the tomato salad ingredients in a bowl. Serve the hot scallops with the tomato salad on the side.

Tomato Salad

3 cups one-inch chunks ripe tomatoes

¼ cup fresh basil leaves, not packed, cut into thin shreds

3 tablespoons balsamic vinegar

1 teaspoon cold-pressed extra-virgin olive oil

Per serving: Calories 249; Total fat: 5g; Saturated fat: 2g; Cholesterol: 72mg; Sodium: 584mg; Carbohydrates: 22g; Fiber: 3g; Sugar: 11g; Protein: 33g.

(Recipe by Annabel Cohen)

Broiled Tilapia with Cucumber Salsa

Prep time: 15 min • **Cook time:** 5 min • **Yield:** 2 servings

Ingredients	Directions
6 ounces boneless and skinless tilapia, cut in half **Sea salt and ground pepper to taste**	**1** Preheat the oven to broil. Spray a rimmed baking sheet with nonstick cooking spray. Arrange the fish on the baking sheet and cook for 5 minutes. **2** While the fish is cooking, combine the salsa ingredients in a medium bowl and stir well. Set aside. **3** Serve the fish, hot, warm, or at room temperature, with the salsa spooned over it. Salt and pepper to taste.

Asian Cucumber Salsa

1 cup seedless cucumber, unpeeled, chopped

2 teaspoons soy sauce

1 tablespoon rice vinegar

1 teaspoon honey

Pinch cayenne pepper to taste

2 tablespoons cilantro, minced

Per serving: Calories 139; Total fat: 3g; Saturated fat: 1g; Cholesterol: 76mg; Sodium: 629mg; Carbohydrates: 5g; Fiber: 1g; Sugar: 5g; Protein: 23g.

(Recipe by Annabel Cohen)

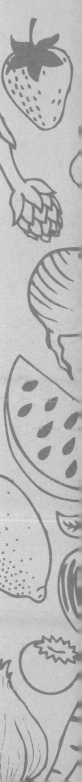

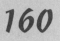

Shrimp and Kelp Noodle Salad

Prep time: 15 min • **Cook time:** None • **Yield:** 2 servings

Ingredients	*Directions*
12 ounces kelp noodles	*1* Rinse the noodles, and then soak them in bowl of water (enough to cover the noodles) and lemon juice and coconut aminos for 3 hours to soften.
2 tablespoons lemon juice	
1 tablespoon coconut aminos	
8 ounces peeled and deveined, cooked, medium-size shrimp (about 15 to 20)	*2* Transfer to a large bowl and add shrimp, the red bell pepper, carrots, snow peas, and scallions. Set aside.
1 cup red bell pepper, cut into thin strips	*3* Combine the dressing ingredients in a small bowl and whisk well. Pour the dressing over the salad and toss well. Add salt and pepper to taste.
½ cup matchstick-cut or shredded carrots	
1 cup snow peas, cut into thin slices	
¼ cup chopped scallions	

Dressing

2 tablespoons rice vinegar

1 teaspoon fresh minced ginger

1 tablespoon coconut aminos

½ to 1 teaspoon ground chili paste to taste

1 tablespoon coconut sugar

1 tablespoon fresh lime juice

Per serving: Calories 229; Total fat: 2g; Saturated fat: 1g; Cholesterol: 182mg; Sodium: 1,254mg; Carbohydrates: 28g; Fiber: 5g; Sugar: 19g; Protein: 22g.

Tip: Kelp noodles don't have the texture of traditional cooked pasta. If you don't soak them, they'll be too crunchy and taste nothing like a noodle. After soaking them, drain well and use.

Tip: Extra low-calorie vegetables, such as shredded Napa cabbage, mung bean sprouts, bok choy, and celery, adds bulk and fiber without the calories.

(Recipe by Annabel Cohen)

Basil and Bell Pepper Shrimp Kebabs

Prep time: 5 min • **Cook time:** 5 min • **Yield:** 2 servings

Ingredients	Directions
8 ounces large, tail-on, peeled, and deveined shrimp **½ red or yellow bell pepper, cut into 6 pieces** **Fresh basil leaves**	**1** Place the shrimp in a medium bowl. Add the marinade ingredients and toss well. Cover and chill for 30 minutes or more.
	2 Preheat the oven to 450°F. Line a rimmed baking sheet with parchment.
	3 Thread four shrimp on each skewer with a piece of bell pepper between each shrimp. Arrange the kebabs on the baking sheet, lightly season with salt and pepper, and cook for 5 minutes. Serve immediately.

Marinade

2 tablespoons fresh basil, chopped

2 tablespoons fresh lemon juice

½ teaspoon grated lemon zest (yellow part only)

½ teaspoon hot pepper sauce (optional)

1 teaspoon cold-pressed extra-virgin olive oil

1 teaspoon fresh thyme, any variety, or ¼ teaspoon dried

Per serving: Calories 137; Total fat: 4g; Saturated fat: 1g; Cholesterol: 182 mg; Sodium: 818mg; Carbohydrates: 4g; Fiber: 1g; Sugar: 2g; Protein: 20g.

Vary It: In addition to the peppers, add slices of onion to the kebabs if desired.

(Recipe by Annabel Cohen)

Tackling Some Pork or Lamb

Pork and lamb in small portions can also provide protein to your diet. Eating protein-rich meats — making sure you trim off any excess fat — and adding a side of vegetables can fill you and make you feel satisfied.

These recipes offer pork for a dinner meal and a breakfast meal. Of course, if you feel like mixing up things, eat the frittata for dinner and the stir fry for your earlier meal. We also include a Greek-inspired lamb tacos recipe here (without the dairy).

Figure 9-3: Trimming away fat from fattier cuts of meat keeps your foods healthier.

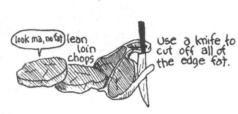

Illustrations by Elizabeth Kurtzman

Quick Pork and Vegetable Stir Fry

Prep time: 30 min • **Cook time:** 10 min • **Yield:** 2 servings

Ingredients	*Directions*
2 teaspoons coconut oil	*1* Add the oil to a large skillet and heat over high heat until hot. Working quickly, add the gingerroot, garlic, and red pepper flakes, and sauté for 10 to 15 seconds.
1 teaspoon minced fresh gingerroot or more to taste	
½ teaspoon minced garlic	
⅛ to ¼ teaspoon red pepper flakes to taste	*2* Add the pork and carrots and sauté for a couple more minutes.
4 ounces pork loin, cut into thin strips	
½ carrot rounds, sliced quarter-inch thick	*3* Add the bean sprouts, asparagus, and bell pepper, and cook until the vegetables are bright and tender-crisp, about 1 to 2 minutes more.
2 cups mung bean sprouts	
3 ounces asparagus, cut into 1-inch diagonal pieces	*4* Stir in the coconut aminos and cook, stirring another minute. Add salt and pepper to taste.
½ small bell pepper, any color, cut into thin strips	
1 tablespoon coconut aminos or more to taste	
Fine sea salt and fresh ground pepper to taste	

Per serving: Calories 165; Total fat: 6g; Saturated fat: 5g; Cholesterol: 30mg; Sodium: 410mg; Carbohydrates: 13g; Fiber: 4g; Sugar: 7g; Protein: 15g.

Vary It: You can also use chicken, turkey, or shrimp instead of the pork, if desired.

Tip: To make this dish vegetarian, double the amounts of vegetables, and eat something else, such as a crisp apple for dessert, to make up the remaining calories.

Tip: Vegetables continue to cook even after you take them out of the hot pan. Don't overcook them. They should be crisp. If you overcook them, they'll become mushy.

(Recipe by Annabel Cohen)

Egg White Prosciutto and Vegetable Frittata

Prep time: 10 min • **Cook time:** 20 mins • **Yield:** 2 servings

Ingredients	Directions
8 egg whites	**1** Preheat the oven to 325°F. Drizzle 1 tablespoon of the olive oil in an large 10-inch nonstick, ovenproof skillet.
2 tablespoons cold-pressed extra-virgin olive oil, separated	
¼ cup chopped onions	**2** Whisk the egg whites in a medium bowl until slightly foamy.
¼ cup chopped zucchini, unpeeled	
1 cup fresh baby spinach, packed	**3** Heat the nonstick skillet (10 to 12 inches) over medium heat until hot. Add the onions, zucchini, and spinach, and sauté until the spinach is wilted and the onions are softened.
½ cup chopped prosciutto	
¼ cup chopped, seeded tomato	**4** Add the prosciutto, tomato, and basil and cook for another minute.
2 tablespoons fresh shredded basil leaves	
2 cups baby arugula	**5** Add the egg whites to the pan over the vegetables. Lightly season with salt and pepper. Cook on top of the stove for 1 minute.
2 to 3 tablespoons balsamic vinegar	
	6 Place the pan in the oven for 10 to 15 minutes until the eggs are set. Remove from the oven and run a spatula around and under the frittata. Tilt the pan to tip the frittata onto a plate. Sprinkle with fresh basil.
	7 Top the frittata with arugula and drizzle with balsamic vinegar and the remaining olive oil.

Per serving: *Calories 311; Total fat: 18g; Saturated fat: 3g; Cholesterol: 28mg; Sodium: 1,204mg; Carbohydrates: 12g; Fiber: 2g; Sugar: 7g; Protein: 27g.*

Tip: You can substitute ⅓ cup frozen chopped spinach for the fresh spinach. Make sure it's thawed and drained well.

(Recipe by Annabel Cohen)

Greek Lamb Tacos

Prep time: 15 min • **Cook time:** 15 min • **Yield:** 2 servings

Ingredients	Directions
1 tablespoon cold-pressed extra-virgin olive oil	*1* Heat the oil in a large nonstick skillet over medium heat. Add the onions and garlic and sauté for 2 minutes. Add the lamb and sauté for 3 more minutes. Add the mint, parsley, sea salt, and pepper, and sauté for another 3 minutes.
2 tablespoons minced onions	
¼ teaspoon minced garlic	
8 ounces very lean ground lamb	
1 tablespoon minced fresh mint	*2* Serve the tacos with the lettuce leaves as taco shells. Top with the tomato and cucumber and add a squeeze of fresh lemon.
1 tablespoon minced fresh parsley	
½ teaspoon fine sea salt	
¼ teaspoon fresh ground pepper	
Romaine lettuce leaves	
1 cup chopped fresh tomato	
1 cup chopped cucumber	
Fresh lemon wedges	

Per serving: Calories 235; Total fat: 13g; Saturated fat: 3g; Cholesterol: 65mg; Sodium: 638mg; Carbohydrates: 7g; Fiber: 3g; Sugar: 4g; Protein: 23g.

Aiming for Meatless Dishes

Every once in a while it's good to go meatless. Not every meal must contain animal products. So many choices are available these days for delicious food options that you won't miss the animal proteins in the following recipes.

And if you're a vegetarian, you can find some creative and tasty options here. Every recipe contains a good source of protein, including nuts, and dark greens, such as kale and mushrooms. Figure 9-4 shows a variety of leafy greens you can eat on the 5:2 Diet.

Here you can find recipes for egg dishes as well as recipes that utilize the pure proteins in egg whites and are bulked with lots of colorful vegetables.

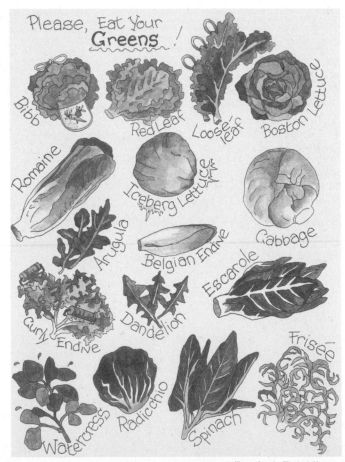

Figure 9-4:
Try a different leafy green each week and see which ones you prefer.

Illustrations by Elizabeth Kurtzman

Spinach Salad with Carrots, Tomatoes, Blueberries, and Honey Mustard Vinaigrette

Prep time: 10 min • **Cook time:** None • **Yield:** 2 servings

Ingredients	Directions
6 cups fresh baby spinach	**1** Combine the spinach, carrots, blueberries, tomatoes, onions, mint, and sunflower seeds in a large bowl.
1 cup shredded carrots	
1 cup fresh blueberries	**2** Whisk together the dressing in another bowl.
8 grape tomatoes, halved lengthwise	
¼ cup minced green onions or scallions	**3** Toss the salad with the dressing and add salt and pepper to taste.
2 tablespoons fresh chopped mint leaves	
2 tablespoons sunflower seeds	
Fine sea salt and fresh ground pepper to taste	

Dressing

3 tablespoons apple cider vinegar	
1 tablespoon cold-pressed extra-virgin olive oil	
1 tablespoon honey	
1 teaspoon grained Dijon mustard	
½ teaspoon minced fresh garlic	

Per serving: *Calories 256; Total fat: 11g; Saturated fat: 1g; Cholesterol: 0mg; Sodium: 513mg; Carbohydrates: 39g; Fiber: 9g; Sugar: 21g; Protein: 6g.*

Tip: Substitute your favorite berries, nuts, and herbs in this recipe to make it your own.

(Recipe by Annabel Cohen)

Dijon Egg White Salad

Prep time: 20 min • **Cook time:** 12 min • **Yield:** 2 servings

Ingredients	*Directions*
8 eggs	*1* Place the eggs in a large saucepan. Add enough cold water to cover the eggs by an inch. Bring to a rapid boil over high heat. Cover and cook for 3 minutes. Remove from the heat and allow to stand for 15 minutes.
1 tablespoon cold-pressed extra-virgin olive oil	
1 tablespoon grained Dijon mustard	
¼ cup chopped celery	*2* Rinse the eggs under cold water and allow them to cool to touch. Roll the eggs on a clean surface to crack the shells, and peel them.
1 cup carrot sticks	
1 medium cucumber sliced	
8 grape tomatoes	*3* Break the eggs apart and remove the yolks. Chop the egg whites on a cutting board with a sharp knife and transfer to a medium bowl. Add the mayo, Dijon mustard, and celery, and fold to mix. Add salt and pepper to taste.
Fine sea salt and fresh ground pepper to taste	
	4 Serve with the carrots, sliced cucumbers, and grape tomatoes on the side for dipping or spreading

Per serving: Calories 196; Total fat: 7g; Saturated fat: 1g; Cholesterol: 0mg; Sodium: 744mg; Carbohydrates: 16g; Fiber: 4g; Sugar: 8g; Protein: 17g.

Note: Figure 9-5 shows how to slice a cucumber.

Note: Dijon mustard has only about 3 calories in each teaspoon, but it can add up. A whole tablespoon can contain up to 10 calories. Check the label to be sure.

(Recipe by Annabel Cohen)

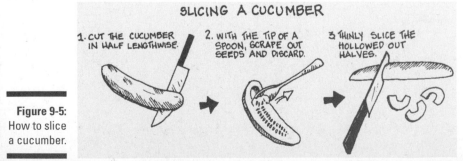

SLICING A CUCUMBER

1. CUT THE CUCUMBER IN HALF LENGTHWISE.
2. WITH THE TIP OF A SPOON, SCRAPE OUT SEEDS AND DISCARD.
3. THINLY SLICE THE HOLLOWED OUT HALVES.

Figure 9-5: How to slice a cucumber.

Illustrations by Elizabeth Kurtzman

Roasted Vegetable Lettuce Sandwiches

Prep time: 15 min • **Cook time:** 15 min • **Yield:** 2 servings

Ingredients	Directions
1 medium bell pepper, any color, cut into 1-inch pieces	**1** Preheat the oven to 450°F. Line a rimmed baking sheet with parchment and set aside.
½ cup carrot circles sliced	**2** Toss the bell peppers, carrots, and onions in a medium bowl with oil. Brush any remaining oil from the bowl over the eggplant. Spread the vegetables on the baking sheet and roast for 10 minutes. Remove the vegetables and roast them for about 5 minutes more until just tender. Remove from the oven and cool completely. Season with salt and pepper to taste.
½ cup sliced onions	
1 small eggplant, cut into 1-inch chunks	
2 teaspoons olive oil	
Fine sea salt and fresh ground pepper to taste	
Balsamic vinegar to taste	**3** Use lettuce leaves to make these sandwiches. Top the vegetables with a spoonful of coconut cream and balsamic vinegar.
Iceberg lettuce leaves	
2 tablespoons coconut cream	
1 tablespoon balsamic vinegar	

Per serving: Calories 184; Total fat: 10g; Saturated fat: 5g; Cholesterol: 0mg; Sodium: 322mg; Carbohydrates: 22g; Fiber: 8g; Sugar: 12g; Protein: 4g.

Note: Figure 9-6 shows how to dice an eggplant.

Vary It: To convert this recipe into a salad, serve the vegetables over a bed of greens, or chop the Romaine lettuce and add 1 cup diced fresh tomatoes or grape or cherry tomatoes.

(Recipe by Annabel Cohen)

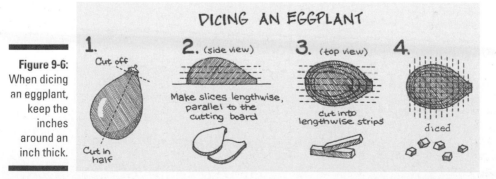

Figure 9-6: When dicing an eggplant, keep the inches around an inch thick.

DICING AN EGGPLANT

1. Cut off / Cut in half
2. (side view) Make slices lengthwise, parallel to the cutting board
3. (top view) cut into lengthwise strips
4. diced

Illustrations by Elizabeth Kurtzman

"Spaghetti" with Eggplant Ragu

Prep time: 40 min • **Cook time:** 60 min • **Yield:** 2 servings

Ingredients	*Directions*
1 whole spaghetti squash	**1** Use a large knife to halve the squash lengthwise through the stem ends. Scoop out the seeds with a spoon. Place the squash halves, cut sides up, on a baking sheet and bake at 375°F for 40 to 50 minutes, or until the squash pierces easily with knife.
¼ cup chopped onions	
½ teaspoon minced garlic	
3 cups peeled eggplant, diced into half-inch pieces	
	2 While the squash is baking, combine all the ragu ingredients in a medium saucepan and bring to a boil over medium-high heat. Reduce heat and simmer for 30 minutes, until the sauce is thickened. Adjust salt and pepper to taste.
	3 Use a fork to scrape out the "spaghetti." Measure two 2-cup servings of the spaghetti and arrange on dinner-sized plates.
	4 Serve the squash with the ragu spooned over.

Ragu

1 cup diced tomatoes in juice

1 cup water

1 tablespoon dried parsley flakes

¼ teaspoon red pepper flakes

Pinch dried oregano

Pinch dried thyme

Fine sea salt and fresh ground pepper to taste

Per serving: Calories 194; Total fat: 2g; Saturated fat: 0g; Cholesterol: 0mg; Sodium: 728mg; Carbohydrates: 46g; Fiber: 13g; Sugar: 20g; Protein: 6g.

(Recipe by Annabel Cohen)

Fresh Fruit Salad with Coconut Cream

Prep time: 15 min • **Cook time:** None • **Yield:** 2 servings

Ingredients	Directions
¼ melon cantaloupe, peeled and cut into 1-inch chunks	**1** Combine all the fruits in two salad bowls. Drizzle with lime juice.
1 cup 1-inch watermelon chunks	
1 cup sliced strawberries	**2** Spoon a tablespoon of coconut cream over each bowl and serve.
1 orange, peeled and divided into sections	
1 apple, unpeeled, cut into 1-inch chunks	
1 tablespoon fresh lime juice	
2 tablespoons coconut cream	

Per serving: Calories 196; Total fat: 6g; Saturated fat: 5g; Cholesterol: 0mg; Sodium: 15mg; Carbohydrates: 42g; Fiber: 9g; Sugar: 31g; Protein: 3g.

Tip: To turn this mixture into a smoothie, combine all the ingredients in a blender with 1 cup of ice. Blend until smooth.

(Recipe by Annabel Cohen)

Chapter 10

For Men: 600-Calorie Meal Recipes

In This Chapter

▶ Knowing what you can eat during your fasting eating window

▶ Discovering easy 600-calorie recipes that are free of grains and dairy

During your fasting period, you'll want to eat meals that are nutritious and delicious. These recipes are geared toward men; at 300 calories (or so) per serving they're healthful and tasty. A few recipes are a tad more than 300 calories per serving, so you'll need to adjust your other meal to stay under 600 calories for the day. Although 300 calories seems like very little when it comes to preparing entrees, with a little imagination, some interesting ingredients, and fresh foods, you can make these meals are easy to prepare and are satisfying and delicious. These protein-rich foods, such as lean beef, poultry, lamb, and pork, trimmed of much fat as possible, promote feelings of feeling full and satisfied for a longer periods of time after eating. Smaller portions of high-quality protein allow you to eat less because lean protein is slower to digest in the body.

These foods are filled with the flavors and textures so many people crave. The high protein content of each recipe means you'll feel fuller than you would if you had eaten hunger-inducing carbohydrates. So, not only will you not starve, you'll eat and feel good about it.

When planning your meals during your eating window, fill up on lean proteins, vegetables, and fruit fiber, and limit calorie-bomb fats and carbohydrates, such as white flour, rice, and sugar. The recipes in this chapter focus on protein from animal and vegetable sources as well as fiber from crunchy vegetables. You can add seasonings, such as fresh and dried herbs, citrus, and the tangy soy-sauce substitute, coconut aminos. (*Coconut aminos* are a soy substitute.)

You can eat them for lunch or dinner, and some are perfect breakfast foods. And nearly all the recipes in this chapter feed two people, so you can either make enough for yourself for two meals or share.

You can easily double or triple these recipes to feed a family just like you can with the recipes in Chapter 9. If you want more bulk to your meal, add a plain green lettuce salad — any lettuce — with a squeeze of fresh lemon juice or vinegar (no oil!).

The ingredients for the recipes here are available in many markets and health-food groceries, so you should have no trouble finding what you need.

> ### Recipes in This Chapter (contd.)
>
> ▶ Kale Salad with Apples and Cherries
> ▶ Squash Soup and Mixed Green Salad with Pears and Walnuts
> ▶ Cream of Mushroom Soup
> ▶ Greek Scramble
> ▶ Eggs in Purgatory
> ▶ Slow-Cooked Pulled Barbecue Pork
> ▶ Slow-Cooked Lamb Chops with Oregano

Creating Some Dishes with Beef

Men can eat 600 calories when fasting on the 5:2 Diet, which can be quite a lot of food, if you're only eating vegetables. But by adding protein-rich foods, such as lean beef, trimmed of as much fat as possible, you're actually going to feel more satisfied for a longer time after eating. Smaller portions of high-quality protein allow you to eat less because lean protein is slower to digest in the body — so that by the time your body digests the beef, you're ready to eat again.

Make sure you eat lean beef. You can ensure that you do so by buying your beef, as well as other meats, poultry, and seafood, from reputable sources.

The following recipes use many different cuts of beef as their main ingredient. The beef is always trimmed as much as possible of visible fat and paired with bulky vegetables and seasoning to make a tasty and nutritious meal. Here we include some salads, a breakfast food, and a couple entrees.

Beef Lettuce Wrap Tacos

Prep time: 15 min • **Cook time:** 15 min • **Yield:** 2 servings

Ingredients	Directions
1 tablespoon cold-pressed extra-virgin olive oil **2 tablespoon minced onions** **¼ teaspoon minced garlic** **1 teaspoon medium chili powder** **6 ounces very lean ground beef** **1 tablespoon minced fresh cilantro** **1 tablespoon minced fresh parsley** **½ teaspoon fine sea salt** **¼ teaspoon fresh ground pepper**	**1** Heat the oil in a large nonstick skillet over medium heat. Add the onions, garlic, and chili powder and sauté for 2 minutes. Add the beef and sauté for another 3 minutes. Add the remaining taco ingredients and sauté for 3 more minutes. **2** Combine the salsa ingredients in a small bowl and mix well. Add salt and pepper to taste. **3** Serve the tacos using the lettuce leaves as "taco shells" and topped with salsa and avocado.

Salsa

½ cup chopped Roma or plum tomatoes

½ cup chopped cucumbers, peeled or unpeeled

1 tablespoon chopped cilantro

1 tablespoon fresh lemon juice

Pinch cayenne pepper

Fine sea salt and fresh ground pepper to taste

Romaine lettuce leaves

1 cup thin sliced fresh avocado

Per serving: Calories 269; Total fat: 18g; Saturated fat: 4g; Cholesterol: 50mg; Sodium: 762mg; Carbohydrates: 13g; Fiber: 8g; Sugar: 3g; Protein: 22g.

(Recipe by Annabel Cohen)

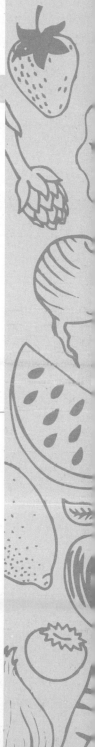

Seared Beef Tenderloin Salad with Garlic Sesame Vinaigrette

Prep time: 30 min • **Cook time:** 20 min • **Yield:** 2 servings

Ingredients	Directions
6 ounces beef tenderloin, uncut	*1* Dry the meat with a paper towel and brush with the melted coconut oil.
1 teaspoon melted coconut oil	
Fine sea salt and ground pepper, to taste	*2* Heat a dry skillet over high heat until very hot. Add the beef and sear until brown on all sides.
2 cups shredded romaine lettuce	*3* Transfer to a cutting board, cover loosely with aluminum foil, and let rest for 5 minutes.
½ cup chopped cucumber	
¼-inch diced tomato	*4* In a small bowl, whisk together the dressing.
2 tablespoons minced red or Bermuda onion	*5* In another large bowl, combine the ingredients and drizzle most of the dressing over the salad.
	6 Arrange the salad on dinner-size plates and top with the beef.
	7 Slice the beef across the grain and serve fanned over the salad. Drizzle remaining dressing over the beef. Season with salt and pepper to serve.

Dressing

2 tablespoons cider vinegar

½ teaspoon minced garlic

1 teaspoon cold-pressed, extra-virgin olive oil

1 teaspoon whole grain mustard

Per serving: Calories 188; Total fat: 10g; Saturated fat: 4g; Cholesterol: 50mg; Sodium: 392mg; Carbohydrates: 5g; Fiber: 2g; Sugar: 2g; Protein: 18g.

Tip: Cook the beef for 4 to 5 minutes total for medium rare.

Grilled Flank Steak with Fresh Mango and Cilantro Salsa

Prep time: 30 min • **Cook time:** 20 min • **Yield:** 2 servings

Ingredients	Directions
8 ounces flank steak	*1* To make the salsa, combine all the salsa ingredients in a medium bowl and stir until uniform. Season with salt and pepper to taste. Chill until ready to serve.
1 teaspoon olive oil	
½ teaspoon fine sea salt	
¼ teaspoon ground cumin	*2* Preheat the grill to medium-high. Rub the beef with olive oil. Season the steak by rubbing with the salt, cumin, pepper, and garlic. Grill the beef for about 8 to 12 minutes on both sides for medium-rare. Remove from the grill and let stand for about 5 minutes.
⅛ teaspoon black pepper	
½ teaspoon granulated garlic	
	3 Holding a knife at a 45-degree angle, slice the steak into thin slices. Spoon the salsa over the beef or serve on the side.

Salsa

½ cup chopped mango

½ cup fresh chopped tomato

2 tablespoons chopped red onion

2 tablespoons chopped fresh cilantro

1–2 tablespoons fresh lemon juice to taste

¼ jalapeño pepper, seeded and minced

Fine sea salt and fresh ground pepper to taste

Per serving: Calories 220; Total fat: 9g; Saturated fat: 3g; Cholesterol: 65mg; Sodium: 920mg; Carbohydrates: 10g; Fiber: 2g; Sugar: 7g; Protein: 24g.

Tip: Wear rubber gloves when seeding and mincing a jalapeño pepper because the juice and seeds can burn. Don't touch your eyes without washing your hands with warm water and soap.

(Recipe by Annabel Cohen)

Meat Lovers' Egg and Vegetable Frittata

Prep time: 20 min • **Cook time:** 30 min • **Yield:** 2 servings

Ingredients	Directions
2 teaspoons coconut oil ¼ cup minced onions	*1* Preheat the oven to 350°F. Cut two sheets of heavy-duty aluminum foil about 14 inches long each.
6 ounces lean (95 percent lean) ground beef 4 slices cooked bacon, crumbled or chopped ½ cup seeded and chopped tomatoes	*2* Heat the oil in a large (10-inch) nonstick skillet over medium-high heat. Add the onions and sauté for a minute. Add the beef and sauté until the meat is cooked through. Add the spinach, bacon, tomatoes, salt, and pepper, and stir for another minute. Transfer the mixture to a dish and set aside.
1 cup frozen, chopped spinach, thawed and very well drained ½ teaspoon salt	*3* Whisk the egg whites in a medium bowl until foamy. Add the whole eggs and whisk until incorporated. Add the meat and vegetable mixture to the eggs and stir to incorporate.
Pinch fresh ground pepper 6 egg whites (about 1 cup)	*4* Spray the skillet well with nonstick cooking spray. Pour the egg mixture into the skillet.
2 eggs	*5* Transfer the skillet to the oven and bake, uncovered, for 20 minutes, until the frittata is set. Use a spatula to loosen the frittata and slide it out of the skillet to a cutting board. Cut the frittata in half and serve.

Per serving: Calories 401; Total fat: 20g; Saturated fat: 10g; Cholesterol: 250mg; Sodium: 1332mg; Carbohydrates: 8g; Fiber: 2g; Sugar: 4g; Protein: 43g.

Vary It!: Add different vegetables to the mix or make it completely vegetarian. If using only vegetables and no meat, you can add more eggs and vegetables to make this omelet really hearty.

(Recipe by Annabel Cohen)

Braised Veal and Mushrooms

Prep time: 10 min • **Cook time:** 15 min • **Yield:** 2 servings

Ingredients	Directions
8 ounces veal scaloppini	*1* Pat the veal skin dry with paper towels and season generously with salt and pepper.
Fine sea salt and fresh ground pepper to taste	
2 teaspoons coconut oil	*2* Heat oil over medium-high heat. Add the veal to the pan and cook it until it's lightly colored. Turn the pieces over and brown them on the other side. Remove the veal to a dish and set aside.
3 sliced cooked bacon, chopped	
½ cup chopped onions	
½ teaspoon minced garlic	*3* Add the bacon, onions, garlic, and red pepper flakes, and sauté until the onions are softened. Add the mushrooms, and sauté for 3 to 4 minutes or until they release their juices. Add the broth, parsley flakes, tomato paste, thyme, and bay leaf to the pan. Bring to a boil and reduce the heat to a simmer. Cook for 5 minutes more.
¼ teaspoon crushed red pepper flakes	
8 ounces sliced mushrooms, any variety	
1 cup fat-free chicken or beef stock or broth	
2 tablespoons dried parsley flakes	*4* Season with salt and pepper to taste in the sauce. Add the veal and heat through, about 2 more minutes. Serve the veal with the sauce spooned over it.
1 tablespoon tomato paste	
1 sprig fresh thyme or ¼ teaspoon dried	
1 bay leaf	

Per serving: Calories 311; Total fat: 13g; Saturated fat: 7g; Cholesterol: 103mg; Sodium: 764mg; Carbohydrates: 12g; Fiber: 3g; Sugar: 4g; Protein: 37g.

Vary It!: You can also use chicken, thin beef steaks, or turkey breast.

(Recipe by Annabel Cohen)

Calling it Fowl: Some Poultry Meals

The protein from skinless and boneless chicken breast meat and turkey breast meat is extremely lean. This lean protein digests slowly in the body, leading to feelings of fullness for longer. White meat, boneless and skinless chicken breast meat, and turkey breast meat boast about 30 calories per ounce, which means that you can eat quite a bit of poultry as part of this very low-calorie staple of your fasting regime. And because the flavor of poultry is mild, it pairs well with so many other ingredients and cooks quickly, which makes it easy to prepare in so many different ways.

The following recipes have flavor and textures. You can find poultry used in fresh salads, stir-fries, roasted choices, and even a meatloaf burger. Each is easy to prepare, yet tastes like restaurant-quality meals.

Living longer: A combination of diet and fasting

The Mediterranean Diet surged in popularity a few years ago and still remains prevalent today. People started to notice that the people who lived in the Mediterranean region seemed to live really long and suffered far less from the common ailments of Western culture. They concluded that those people must have lived longer because of their diet. So now many people sprinkle extra virgin olive oil on everything with the hopes that it will add years to their life. (Extra-virgin olive oil is very good for you, no doubt, and so are many other elements of Mediterranean cuisine, particularly seafood.)

However, although this diet certainly does contribute to their longevity, it may not be the whole truth. For example, look at the region of Crete. The Cretan population is celebrated for its excellent health and longevity. But what about Crete makes it stand out amongst other regions in the Mediterranean?

The answer, of course, is in part their fresh and simple diet. But the other part, the lesser-known part, is fasting. Although fasting is mostly a religious practice for people who live on Crete, the positive health effects can't be denied. For many years scientists have studied the fasting rituals of the Greek Orthodox Christian Church. The evidence is indisputable: Fasting and their Mediterranean eating habits largely attributes to the robust health of the Cretan population.

Club Salad

Prep time: 20 min • **Cook time:** 10 min • **Yield:** 2 servings

Ingredients	Directions
1 cup cubed cooked boneless and skinless chicken breast	*1* Combine the salad ingredients in a bowl.
2 strips cooked bacon, chopped or crumbled	*2* Combine the dressing ingredients in a small bowl and whisk well. Set aside.
1 cup tomatoes, chopped, or grape tomatoes, halved	*3* Add the dressing to the salad and toss well.
½ cup shredded or grated carrots	
2 tablespoons chopped red onion	
3 cups chopped romaine lettuce	

Dressing

2 tablespoons cold-pressed, extra-virgin olive oil

1 teaspoon dried dill

¼ teaspoon granulated garlic

2 teaspoons fresh lemon juice

¼ teaspoon hot pepper sauce

Fine sea salt and fresh ground black pepper to taste

Per serving: *Calories 268; Total fat: 18g; Saturated fat: 4g; Cholesterol: 90mg; Sodium: 478mg; Carbohydrates: 10g; Fiber: 4g; Sugar: 5g; Protein: 24g.*

(Recipe by Annabel Cohen)

Chicken Lettuce Wraps

Prep time: 10 min • **Cook time:** 15 min • **Yield:** 2 servings

Ingredients	*Directions*
1 tablespoon coconut oil	**1** Heat a skillet over medium-high heat until hot. Add all onions and sauté for 2 minutes. Add the remaining ingredients and sauté until hot.
8 ounces cooked (boiled, baked, or grilled) boneless and skinless chicken breasts, chopped	
½ cup chopped onions	**2** Serve with lettuce leaves and extra coconut aminos if desired.
½ cup water chestnuts	
2 tablespoons coconut aminos	
2 teaspoons coconut sugar	
2 teaspoons fresh lime juice	
1 teaspoon grated fresh ginger	
½ teaspoon minced garlic	
Pinch red pepper flakes	
Iceberg lettuce leaves	

Per serving: Calories 312; Total fat: 11g; Saturated fat: 7g; Cholesterol: 96mg; Sodium: 431mg; Carbohydrates: 16g; Fiber: 2g; Sugar: 8g; Protein: 36g.

Note: Canned water chestnuts are okay to use.

(Recipe by Annabel Cohen)

Chicken, Mushroom, and Vegetable Stir Fry

Prep time: 30 min • **Cook time:** 10 min • **Yield:** 2 servings

Ingredients	Directions
2 teaspoons coconut oil	*1* Add 1 teaspoon coconut oil to a large skillet and heat over high heat until hot. Working quickly, add the ginger, garlic, and red pepper flakes and sauté for 30 seconds to a minute.
1 teaspoon minced fresh ginger, or more to taste	
½ teaspoon minced garlic	
⅛ to ¼ teaspoon red pepper flakes to taste	*2* Add the chicken and sauté for 2 more minutes.
6 ounces boneless and skinless chicken breast, cut into 1-inch chunks	*3* Add the mushrooms and sauté for 2 more minutes. Remove the chicken and mushrooms to a dish and set aside.
8 ounces button mushrooms, rinsed	
1 cup shredded cabbage	*4* Add another teaspoon of the coconut oil to the skillet and add the shredded cabbage, carrot rounds, celery, and bell pepper. Sauté for 2 minutes or until the vegetables are bright and tender-crisp.
½ cup carrot rounds, sliced quarter-inch think	
½ cup chopped celery	*5* Stir in the coconut aminos and cook, stirring 1 more minute. Don't overcook; you want the vegetables to be very crisp. Add the chicken and mushrooms back to the skillet and heat through. Add salt and pepper to taste and sprinkle with sesame seeds and serve.
½ small bell pepper, any color, cut into thin strips	
1 tablespoon coconut aminos or more to taste	
Fine sea salt and fresh ground pepper to taste	
1 teaspoon sesame seeds, any color	

Per serving: *Calories 213; Total fat: 8g; Saturated fat: 5g; Cholesterol: 47mg; Sodium: 671mg; Carbohydrates: 14g; Fiber: 4g; Sugar: 4g; Protein: 23g.*

Tip: Vegetables continue to cook even after you take them out of the hot pan. If you cook them too long, they'll become mushy.

(Recipe by Annabel Cohen)

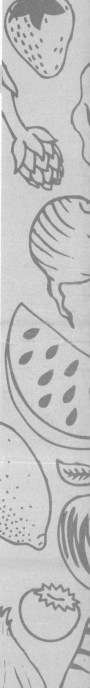

Spicy Maple-Grilled Chicken and Vegetables

Prep time: 15 min • **Cook time:** 40 min • **Yield:** 2 servings

Ingredients	Directions
8 ounces boneless and skinless chicken breast	*1* Heat the grill to medium-high. Combine all the basting ingredients in a bowl and whisk well. Set aside half of the sauce in another bowl.
1 teaspoon olive oil	
½ pound peeled carrots, cut in half, lengthwise	*2* Brush the chicken with oil and place on the hot grill. Brush with basting sauce and grill on both sides until the chicken is cooked through, about 8 to 12 minutes.
1 small eggplant, sliced into half-inch slices, lengthwise	
½ pound asparagus (tough ends removed) or zucchini (cut the zucchini into thick slices)	*3* Spray the vegetables lightly with nonstick cooking spray. After adding the chicken to the grill, add the raw vegetables to the grill, and grill until the vegetables are just cooked through (don't overcook).
½ Spanish onion, quartered	*4* Remove from the grill and cut the carrots and eggplant into bite-sized pieces. Arrange the vegetables on a serving platter and serve them with the chicken. Drizzle the reserved basting sauce over the chicken and vegetables.

Basting Sauce

¼ cup chopped onion

1 teaspoon minced garlic

½ teaspoon red pepper flakes

1 tablespoon coconut aminos

1 tablespoon apple cider vinegar

1 tablespoon maple syrup

½ teaspoon allspice

Pinch of dried thyme

Pinch ground cloves

¼ teaspoon cinnamon

Per serving: Calories 293; Total fat: 5g; Saturated fat: 1g; Cholesterol: 63mg; Sodium: 325mg; Carbohydrates:35 g; Fiber: 9g; Sugar: 21g; Protein: 28g.

Vary It!: Use any vegetables you desire in this dish.

(Recipe by Annabel Cohen)

Chicken Tikka Masala

Prep time: 30 min • **Cook time:** 40 min • **Yield:** 2 servings

Ingredients	*Directions*
½ **pound boneless and skinless chicken breasts, visible fat removed**	*1* Cut the chicken into 1-inch chunks. Set aside. Heat the ghee in a saucepan over medium-high heat.
1 **tablespoon ghee**	*2* Add the chicken, onion, garlic, spices, and coconut sugar, and cook until the vegetables are softened, about 5 minutes.
½ **cup finely chopped onion**	
¼ **teaspoon minced garlic**	
¼ **teaspoon ground cumin**	*3* Stir in the tomato sauce and bring to a boil. Add the chicken and coconut milk and lemon juice and stir to combine. Reduce the heat to simmer and cook until hot. Add additional salt and pepper to taste.
¼ **teaspoon curry powder**	
¼ **teaspoon salt**	
¼ **teaspoon ground ginger**	
¼ **teaspoon ground cinnamon**	*4* Serve garnished with fresh cilantro.
Pinch ground black pepper	
Pinch ground turmeric	
Pinch ground cayenne pepper, to taste	
½ **teaspoon paprika**	
1 **teaspoon coconut sugar**	
½ **cup tomato sauce**	
¼ **cup coconut milk**	
1 **tablespoon lemon juice**	
Fresh chopped cilantro	

Per serving: *Calories 290; Total fat: 16g; Saturated fat: 11g; Cholesterol: 83mg; Sodium: 673mg; Carbohydrates: 12g; Fiber: 2g; Sugar: 7g; Protein: 25g.*

(Recipe by Annabel Cohen)

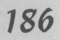

"Buttery" Lemon Chicken

Prep time: 10 min • **Cook time:** 15 min • **Yield:** 2 servings

Ingredients	*Directions*
8 ounces boneless, skinless chicken breast halves	**1** Pound slightly the chicken breasts to make them more or less the same thickness throughout. If the breasts are large, butterfly by slicing through them horizontally to make 2 halves for each breast half.
¼ cup coconut flour for dredging chicken	**2** Place the flour in a medium bowl or on a plate. Dredge the chicken pieces in the flour and coat well. Pat the breasts to remove excess flour.
2 tablespoons ghee or old-pressed, extra-virgin olive oil for sautéing chicken	
1 cup fat-free chicken broth	**3** Heat the ghee or oil in a large nonstick skillet over medium-high heat. Sauté the chicken breasts on each side until they're light golden.
1 tablespoon drained capers	
Fine sea salt and fresh ground pepper to taste	**4** Pour the chicken broth over the chicken and cook until the sauce is reduced and makes a thickened sauce. Adjust the salt and pepper in the sauce to taste.
Juice of up to 1 lemon	**5** Stir in the lemon juice and serve right away. Garnish the chicken with capers and freshly chopped parsley.
¼ cup chopped parsley	

Per serving: *Calories 335; Total fat:19g; Saturated fat: 12g; Cholesterol: 103mg; Sodium: 727mg; Carbohydrates: 11g; Fiber: 5g; Sugar: 2g; Protein:28g.*

Vary It!: Use turkey cutlets or veal cut into scallopini instead of chicken for variety.

(Recipe by Annabel Cohen)

Turkey Meatloaf Burgers

Prep time: 15 min • **Cook time:** 15 min • **Yield:** 2 servings

Ingredients	Directions
12 ounces ground turkey breast meat	**1** Combine the turkey, egg whites, onion, tomato sauce, garlic, oregano, black pepper, and salt in a bowl, and mash with your hands. Form into two burgers.
2 egg whites, lightly beaten	
¼ cup finely chopped onion	**2** Grill over medium-high heat or bake at 450°F on a baking sheet until cooked through, about 12 minutes.
3 tablespoons tomato sauce	
2 garlic cloves, minced	**3** Serve between 2 lettuce leaves as buns and garnish with bell peppers, tomato slices, and mustard.
¼ teaspoon dried oregano	
Pinch fresh ground black pepper	
¼ teaspoon fine sea salt	
Iceberg lettuce leaves	
Red, yellow, or green bell pepper rings	
2 large slices fresh tomato	
Dijon mustard	

Per serving: *Calories 229; Total fat: 11g; Saturated fat: 1g; Cholesterol: 112mg; Sodium: 540mg; Carbohydrates: 7g; Fiber: 2g; Sugar: 4g; Protein: 45g.*

Tip: These burgers are big. In order to bake or grill them, you'll need to make sure they're about 1½-inches thick.

(Recipe by Annabel Cohen)

Jalapeño Chunky Turkey and Veggie Chili

Prep time: 30 min • **Cook time:** 1 hour • **Yield:** 2 servings

Ingredients	Directions
8 ounces ground turkey breast	*1* In a large saucepan, brown the turkey over medium-high heat, stirring often to break up lumps.
1 cup water	
1 can (14.5 ounces) diced tomatoes with juice	*2* Add the water, tomatoes, carrots, celery, onions, chili powder, garlic, cumin, salt, pepper, and jalapeño. Bring to a boil, reduce the heat to simmer, cover, and cook for 30 minutes more.
½ cup quarter-inch diced carrots	
¼ cup chopped celery	*3* Add salt and pepper to taste and serve hot, garnished with scallions.
¼ chopped onions	
2 teaspoons medium chili powder	
1 tablespoon minced garlic	
¾ teaspoon ground cumin	
1 teaspoon fine sea salt	
½ teaspoon ground pepper	
1 teaspoon minced jalapeño pepper or more to taste	
2 tablespoons chopped scallions	

Per serving: Calories 207; Total fat: 1g; Saturated fat: 0g; Cholesterol: 75mg; Sodium: 1,898mg; Carbohydrates: 19g; Fiber: 5g; Sugar: 8g; Protein: 30g.

Vary It!: Substitute beef (very lean) for the turkey in this dish.

(Recipe by Annabel Cohen)

Turkey "Spaghetti" with Ragu

Prep time: 40 min • **Cook time:** 60 min • **Yield:** 2 servings

Ingredients	Directions
1 whole (around 3 pounds) spaghetti squash	**1** Place the squash on a baking sheet and bake at 375°F for 40 to 50 minutes, or until the squash pierces easily with knife.
1 tablespoon ghee	
8 ounces lean ground turkey	**2** While the squash is baking, melt the butter in a saucepan over medium-high heat. Add the turkey and cook, stirring frequently, until almost cooked through, about 3 minutes. Add the onions and garlic and sauté for 2 more minutes.
¾ cup chopped onions	
½ teaspoon minced garlic	
1 can (14.5 ounces) diced tomatoes with juice	**3** Add the remaining ingredients and bring to a boil over medium-high heat. Reduce the heat and simmer for 30 minutes, until the sauce is thickened. Adjust the salt and pepper to taste.
2 tablespoons tomato paste	
½ cup fat-free chicken broth	
¼ tablespoon dried oregano	**4** Halve the squash and carefully spoon out the seeds. Use a fork to scrape out the "spaghetti." Measure two 2½-cup servings of the spaghetti squash and arrange on dinner-size plates.
½ teaspoon dried thyme	
½ teaspoon fine sea salt	
¼ teaspoon cracked black pepper	**5** Serve with the warmed sauce spooned over the spaghetti squash and with additional salt and pepper to taste.

Per serving: Calories 320; Total fat: 4g; Saturated fat: 2g; Cholesterol: 45mg; Sodium: 1,251mg; Carbohydrates: 57g; Fiber: 12g; Sugar: 24g; Protein: 36g.

(Recipe by Annabel Cohen)

Surfing with Seafood Dishes

Seafood and fish are increasingly popular, low-calorie food when you compare them to other protein-rich foods like meat and poultry. Many lean fish varieties contain similar calories per ounce as lean poultry, about 30 to 35 calories. Just make sure that you purchase seafood and fish, preferably as fresh as possible, from a reputable source. Lean fish is also low in both total fat and saturated fat; as a general rule, the lighter the fish, the leaner it is.

Theses recipes include salads, stews, and roasted and grilled fish and shellfish.

Apple, Crab, and Pecan Salad

Prep time: 15 min • **Cook time:** 5 min • **Yield:** 2 servings

Ingredients	Directions
12 ounces canned lump crabmeat	*1* Pick through the crab for any possible shell fragments. Place all the ingredients in a bowl and stir gently until combined.
2 cups diced, unpeeled Granny Smith apple	
¼ cup chopped pecans, lightly toasted	
¼ cup chopped scallions	
¼ cup fresh chopped dill	
2 tablespoons fresh lemon juice	
Fine sea salt and fresh ground pepper, to taste	

Per serving: Calories 335; Total fat: 17g; Saturated fat: 2g; Cholesterol: 165mg; Sodium: 742mg; Carbohydrates: 26g; Fiber: 7g; Sugar: 17g; Protein: 26g.

Vary It!: You can use lobster meat, steamed shrimp, or canned albacore white tuna instead of the crab.

Tip: Serve the crab salad on a bed of greens with additional lemon juice drizzled over.

(Recipe by Annabel Cohen)

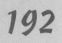

Cod with Olives and Tomatoes

Prep time: 15 min • **Cook time:** 30 min • **Yield:** 2 servings

Ingredients	Directions
1 tablespoon olive oil	**1** Heat the oil in a large nonstick skillet over medium-high heat.
½ cup chopped onion	
1 teaspoon minced garlic	**2** Add the onions, garlic, and bell pepper, and sauté until softened. Add the oregano, olives, cinnamon, tomatoes, parsley, and water, and bring to a boil.
½ chopped bell pepper	
1 teaspoon dried oregano	
2 tablespoon chopped, pitted green olives	**3** Reduce the heat and cook until the flavors are well combined, about 10 minutes, stirring occasionally. Add salt and pepper to taste.
½ teaspoon ground cinnamon	
1 cup chopped fresh tomatoes, any variety	**4** Arrange the fish in a large skillet, spoon the sauce over it, cover with a lid, and cook 4 to 5 minutes, until the fish flakes with a fork. Serve hot.
¼ cup chopped parsley	
½ cup water	
Kosher salt and fresh ground pepper, to taste	
½ pound cod, cut into 2 pieces	

Per serving: Calories 212; Total fat: 10g; Saturated fat: 1g; Cholesterol: 43mg; Sodium: 533mg; Carbohydrates: 12g; Fiber: 3g; Sugar: 5g; Protein: 20g.

Vary It!: Use 6 ounces of chicken or turkey breast meat instead of the fish, if desired. If you do, don't add the green olives.

(Recipe by Annabel Cohen)

Citrus Ginger Salmon with Kale Chips

Prep time: 40 min • **Cook time:** 50 min • **Yield:** 2 servings

Ingredients	*Directions*
Juice of one orange	*1* Combine the orange juice, zest, lime juice, ginger, coconut sugar, and hot pepper sauce in a medium bowl and whisk well. Add the salmon and turn several times in the glaze. Cover and chill for 30 minutes.
¼ teaspoon grated orange zest	
2 teaspoons fresh lime juice	
1 teaspoon minced fresh ginger	*2* To make the kale chips, preheat the oven to 350°F. Line a rimmed baking sheet with parchment paper. With a knife or kitchen shears carefully remove the flakes from the thick stems and tear into bite-size pieces. Wash and thoroughly dry kale with a salad spinner. Drizzle the kale with oil and sprinkle with the seasoning salt. Bake until the edges are brown but aren't burnt, about 10 to 15 minutes. Cool completely before serving.
1 teaspoon coconut sugar	
¼ teaspoon hot pepper sauce	
8 ounces boneless and skinless salmon fillet, cut into two portions	
	3 To prepare the salmon, preheat the oven to 450°F. Line a rimmed baking sheet with parchment paper. Remove the salmon from the refrigerator and place the salmon fillets on the prepared baking sheet. Discard the marinade.
	4 Cook for 7 to 10 minutes. (Don't overcook.) Serve hot, with the kale chips on the side.

Kale Chips

1 bunch kale	
1 tablespoon coconut or olive oil	
1 teaspoon salt	

Per serving: *Calories 265; Total fat: 13g; Saturated fat: 7g; Cholesterol: 53mg; Sodium: 836mg; Carbohydrates: 13g; Fiber: 2g; Sugar: 5g; Protein: 27g.*

Tip: Watch the kale chips as they bake so that they don't get browned and bitter.

(Recipe by Annabel Cohen)

Pesto Roasted Tilapia and Sweet Potato Fries

Prep time: 10 min • **Cook time:** 30 min • **Yield:** 2 servings

Ingredients	Directions
8 ounces tilapia (about 2 fillets)	*1* To prepare the potatoes, preheat the oven to 400°F. Line a rimmed baking sheet with parchment paper.
1 large sweet potato, about 8 ounces, cut into thin wedges	*2* In a large bowl, toss together the potatoes and oil until the potatoes are evenly coated with oil. Lightly season with salt and pepper.
2 teaspoons olive oil	
Fine sea salt and fresh ground pepper to taste	*3* Place the potatoes in a single layer on the baking sheet and bake for about 20 minutes, or until the potatoes are tender and browned. Line another baking sheet with parchment paper and place the fish fillets on it.
	4 Combine the pesto ingredients in a food processor and pulse until almost smooth. Brush half of the pesto over the fish and bake for 10 minutes. Serve the fish with the sweet potatoes on the side and the remaining pesto as a dipping sauce for the fries.

Pesto

½ cup packed fresh arugula

½ cup fresh basil leaves

1 small garlic clove

4 teaspoons extra-virgin olive oil

2 teaspoons fresh lemon juice

Per serving: Calories 307; Total fat: 16g; Saturated fat: 3g; Cholesterol: 76mg; Sodium: 637mg; Carbohydrates: 18g; Fiber: 3g; Sugar: 5g; Protein: 24g.

Tip: Save an extra 10 minutes of cooking time by cooking the fish at the same time as the sweet potato.

(Recipe by Annabel Cohen)

Scallops with Spinach, Grape Tomatoes, and Roasted Parsnips

Prep time: 20 min • **Cook time:** 30 min • **Yield:** 2 servings

Ingredients	Directions
1½ cups (about 6 ounces) peeled, 1-inch cubed parsnips	**1** Preheat the oven to 400°F. Line a rimmed baking sheet with nonstick cooking spray.
1 teaspoon coconut oil, melted	
Fine sea salt to taste	**2** Combine the parsnips and melted coconut oil in a medium bowl and toss well. Spread the parsnips on the prepared baking sheet and season lightly with salt. Bake for 15 to 20 minutes, until just tender. While the parsnips are cooking, dry the scallops with a paper towel. Melt the coconut oil in a large skillet over high heat. Add the scallops and sear for approximately 2 minutes on each side. Transfer the scallops to a dish and set aside.
1 pound bay scallops	
2 teaspoons coconut oil	
1 teaspoon minced garlic	
5 ounces baby spinach leaves	
1 pint grape tomatoes	**3** Add the garlic and spinach to the pan, cover with a lid, and cook for 2 minutes. Transfer the spinach to a bowl and set aside. Add the tomatoes to the pan and sauté for another minute. Season the tomatoes with salt and pepper. Add the scallops back to the pan and heat for another minute.
Paprika to taste	
1 tablespoon chopped parsley	
Fresh lemon wedges, garnish	**4** Serve the scallops with the spinach, tomatoes, and parsnips on the side. Garnish with the paprika and parsley and a lemon wedge.

Per serving: Calories 476; Total fat: 10g; Saturated fat: 6g; Cholesterol: 132mg; Sodium: 1,050mg; Carbohydrates: 42g; Fiber: 9g; Sugar: 9g; Protein: 59g.

(Recipe by Annabel Cohen)

Savory Fish Stew

Prep time: 10 min • **Cook time:** 25 min • **Yield:** 2 servings

Ingredients	*Directions*
2 teaspoons olive oil ½ cup chopped onions	*1* Combine the oil, onions, and garlic in a pot over medium-high heat. Sauté until tender.
½ teaspoon minced garlic One 14-ounce can diced tomatoes in juice	*2* Add the tomatoes, carrots, celery, wine, saffron, zest, and red pepper flakes. Bring to a boil.
¼ cup diced carrots ¼ cup diced celery ½ cup white wine or water	*3* Reduce the heat and cook for 10 minutes more. Add the fish, salt, and pepper. Cover and cook for 10 more minutes. Add half the parsley and adjust the salt and pepper to taste.
Pinch of saffron (optional) ¼ teaspoon grated lemon zest Pinch dried red pepper flakes	*4* Serve sprinkled with the remaining parsley.
½ pound fish: cod, salmon, or snapper fillets are good choices, cut into 2-inch pieces	
Fine sea salt and fresh ground pepper, to taste	
2 tablespoons chopped fresh parsley	

Per serving: Calories 195; Total fat: 5g; Saturated fat: 1g; Cholesterol: 43mg; Sodium: 967mg; Carbohydrates: 16g; Fiber: 3g; Sugar: 8g; Protein: 20g.

(Recipe by Annabel Cohen)

Cooking Some Meatless Meals

You may want a lighter-feeling meal without meat. You can go meatless while on a fasting regimen. In fact, not every meal that you eat must contain animal products.

And if you're a vegetarian, going meatless is clearly your only option. Many delicious food options are available these days. These recipes have protein in the form of nuts, fruits, and dark greens, such as kale and mushrooms. Figure 10-1 shows some types of nuts that these recipes have. You can experiment and substitute your nut preferences. Just remember: Nuts pack on the calories, so use them sparingly.

Here you can find recipes for hearty salads, tasty soups, and egg dishes that utilize the pure proteins in egg whites. These recipes are bulked with lots of colorful vegetables.

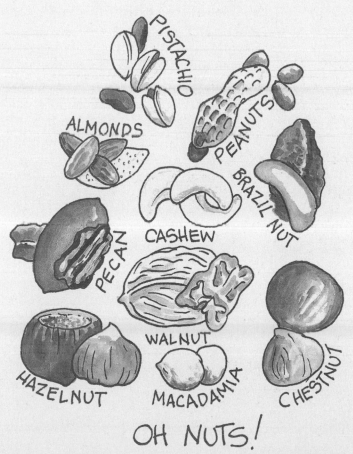

Figure 10-1:
Go nuts!

Illustrations by Elizabeth Kurtzman

Kale Salad with Apples and Cherries

Prep time: 20 min • **Cook time:** None • **Yield:** 2 servings

Ingredients	*Directions*
1 bunch Tuscan kale or regular kale (about a half pound) ½ cup chopped parsley	*1* Wash and dry the kale. Cut away the leaves from the center stems and massage the leaves in your hand by scrunching them until they're softened and dark green.
1 cup quarter-inch diced apples	
½ cup fresh pitted cherries, lightly toasted	*2* Chop the kale and transfer it to a large bowl.
¼ cup shaved red onion	*3* Add the remaining salad ingredients.
Fine sea salt and fresh ground pepper to taste	*4* Combine the dressing ingredients in a small bowl and whisk well.
	5 Pour the dressing over the salad and toss the salad. Allow the salad to rest for 1 hour or more before serving.

Dressing

1 tablespoon white balsamic vinegar

2 tablespoons fresh lemon juice

1 tablespoon extra-virgin olive oil

2 teaspoons honey

1 teaspoon sesame seeds

Per serving: Calories 210; Total fat: 9g; Saturated fat: 1g; Cholesterol: 0mg; Sodium: 331mg; Carbohydrates: 33g; Fiber: 5g; Sugar: 21g; Protein: 4g.

Note: To lightly toast cherries, heat in an oven at 325°F for about 15 minutes.

Tip: The longer the salad rests, the softer and darker green it becomes.

(Recipe by Annabel Cohen)

Squash Soup and Mixed Green Salad with Pears and Walnuts

Prep time: 30 min • **Cook time:** 1.5 hours • **Yield:** 2 servings

Ingredients	Directions
1 tablespoon ghee or olive oil	**1** Prepare the soup first, by melting the ghee in a large saucepan over medium-high heat. Add the onions and cook, stirring for about 3 minutes until the onions are softened.
1 cup chopped onions	
1 pound peeled, cubed winter squash, seeds removed	
2 cups fat-free chicken broth, vegetable broth, or water	**2** Add the squash, broth, nutmeg, salt, and pepper, and bring the soup to a boil. Reduce the heat, cover, and cook for 35 to 40 minutes or until the squash is very tender.
¼ teaspoon nutmeg	
Fine sea salt and fresh ground pepper, to taste	**3** Let the soup cool slightly and transfer some of the soup to a food processor or a blender, or use an immersion blender to puree the soup until very smooth. Repeat with remaining soup. Add additional salt and pepper to taste. Serve hot.
	4 To make the salad, combine the salad ingredients and dressing in a large bowl and toss well.

Salad

4 cups mixed baby greens

¼ cup walnuts

1 cup diced, unpeeled pears

2 tablespoons balsamic vinegar

1 tablespoon cold-pressed extra-virgin olive oil

Per serving: Calories 405; Total fat: 21g; Saturated fat: 6g; Cholesterol: 15mg; Sodium: 756mg; Carbohydrates: 49g; Fiber: 13g; Sugar:18g; Protein: 12g.

Tip: Cook the squash until very soft. This step is very important; if the squash isn't very soft, the soup won't puree smoothly.

Note: Acorn or butternut squash are good choices.

(Recipe by Annabel Cohen)

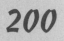

Cream of Mushroom Soup

Prep time: 40 min • **Cook time:** 1 hour • **Yield:** 2 servings

Ingredients	Directions
1 tablespoon coconut oil 1 cup chopped onions 1 teaspoon minced garlic 16 ounces sliced button or white mushrooms 1 teaspoon fresh thyme leaves 3 cups fat-free chicken broth ½ cup canned coconut milk Fine sea salt and fresh ground pepper, to taste	*1* Heat the oil in a large saucepan and add the onions and garlic. Cook, stirring, for 3 minutes. *2* Add the mushrooms, thyme, and chicken broth, and bring to a boil. Reduce the heat and simmer for 20 minutes. *3* Whisk in the coconut milk and cook for 20 minutes more. Add the salt and pepper to taste and cook for 10 minutes more. *4* Serve hot.

Per serving: Calories 320; Total fat: 30g; Saturated fat: 18g; Cholesterol: 0mg; Sodium: 970mg; Carbohydrates: 14g; Fiber: 6g; Sugar: 8g; Protein: 22g

Greek Scramble

Prep time: 5 min • **Cook time:** 10 min • **Yield:** 2 servings

Ingredients	Directions
1 tablespoon ghee or olive oil	**1** Melt the ghee in a large nonstick skillet over medium-heat.
½ cup chopped onions	
3 cups fresh baby spinach	**2** Add the onions and sauté for 5 minutes. Add the baby spinach and sauté until wilted. Add the eggs and scramble for 1 minute. Add the remaining ingredients and scramble for another couple of minutes or so, to your desired doneness.
6 egg whites combined with 2 whole eggs, lightly beaten	
1 cup chopped tomatoes	
¼ cup chopped, pitted kalamata olives	
Fine sea salt and pepper to taste	

Per serving: Calories 263; Total fat: 15g; Saturated fat: 6g; Cholesterol: 201mg; Sodium: 835mg; Carbohydrates: 14g; Fiber: 4g; Sugar: 5g; Protein: 20g.

Note: Figure 10-2 shows how to pit olives.

(Recipe by Annabel Cohen)

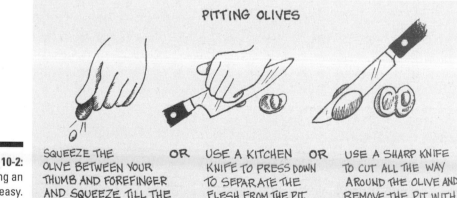

PITTING OLIVES

Figure 10-2: Pitting an olive is easy.

SQUEEZE THE OLIVE BETWEEN YOUR THUMB AND FOREFINGER AND SQUEEZE TILL THE PIT COMES OUT.

OR

USE A KITCHEN KNIFE TO PRESS DOWN TO SEPARATE THE FLESH FROM THE PIT.

OR

USE A SHARP KNIFE TO CUT ALL THE WAY AROUND THE OLIVE AND REMOVE THE PIT WITH YOUR FINGER.

Illustrations by Elizabeth Kurtzman

Eggs in Purgatory

Prep time: 10 min • **Cook time:** 30 min • **Yield:** 2 servings

Ingredients	Directions
1 tablespoon extra-virgin olive oil	*1* Heat the oil in a large skillet over medium-high heat.
½ cup chopped onions	*2* Add the onions and garlic and cook until the onions are tender and golden.
1 teaspoon minced garlic	
One can (14.5 ounces) diced tomatoes with juice	*3* Reduce the heat to simmer. Add the tomatoes, season lightly with salt and pepper, and cook until the tomatoes start to break down, about 20 minutes.
Fresh sea salt and ground pepper, to taste	
3 tablespoons fresh chopped basil	*4* Stir in the basil and taste the sauce, adding more salt and pepper to taste.
4 eggs	
	5 With a spoon, make a well in the center of the tomato sauce. Crack the eggs into the well, cover with a lid, and cook for 3 to 4 minutes, until the egg whites have set but the yolk is runny.
	6 Serve the eggs immediately with the sauce spooned over them.

Per serving: Calories 222; Total fat: 16g; Saturated fat: 4g; Cholesterol: 372mg; Sodium: 434mg; Carbohydrates: 5g; Fiber: 1g; Sugar: 2g; Protein: 13g.

Tip: You can serve this dish for breakfast, lunch, and even dinner, as it is done in Italy.

Note: In essence, eggs cracked into a flavorful tomato sauce are poached in the liquid. You can also scramble the eggs in the sauce. Figure 10-3 demonstrates how to mince garlic.

(Recipe by Annabel Cohen)

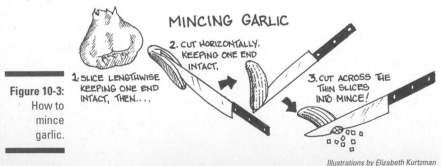

MINCING GARLIC

1. SLICE LENGTHWISE KEEPING ONE END INTACT, THEN....

2. CUT HORIZONTALLY. KEEPING ONE END INTACT.

3. CUT ACROSS THE THIN SLICES INTO MINCE!

Figure 10-3: How to mince garlic.

Illustrations by Elizabeth Kurtzman

Cooking Some Pork and Lamb Cuisine

Pork and lamb often get a bad rap for being fatty and caloric, when in fact, some cuts, such as lean (trimmed of visible fat) pork loin, has nearly the same calories as lean poultry or fish. With less than 40 calories per ounce, lean pork is as versatile as chicken, but with a meaty flavor and texture, as with beef. Of course, as with beef, there are fatty cuts of pork and lamb, which are better left out of a very low-calorie regime. As with all protein choices, the key to eating any meat is the word *lean*. Make sure you buy your pork and lamb from a reputable source.

Like beef, the protein in lamb and pork products is located in the muscle tissue. This lean protein digests slowly in the body, leading to feelings of fullness for longer.

The following recipes include two slow-cooked meals — a delicious pulled pork entree and a tasty lamb chop meal.

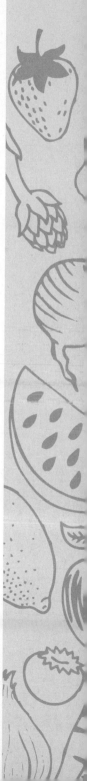

Slow-Cooked Pulled Barbecue Pork

Prep time: 15 min • **Cook time:** 6 hours • **Yield:** 4 servings

Ingredients	Directions
1 pound pork butt	**1** Place all the ingredients in a slow cooker. Cover and cook on low until the pork is very tender, about 6 hours.
1½ cups water	
1 cup tomato sauce	
1 tablespoon minced garlic	**2** Shred the pork by pulling the meat apart with two forks. Add with salt and pepper to taste.
1 teaspoon whole grain Dijon mustard	
1 teaspoon paprika	
1 teaspoon salt	
¼ cup fresh lemon juice	
1 tablespoon honey	

Per serving: Calories 127; Total fat: 4g; Saturated fat: 1g; Cholesterol: 39mg; Sodium: 976mg; Carbohydrates: 10g; Fiber: 1g; Sugar: 7g; Protein: 13g.

Tip: To make into sandwiches, take two pieces of iceberg leaf lettuce and create a "bun."

Tip: This dish freezes well, so you can double or triple the recipe and freeze the rest.

(Recipe by Annabel Cohen)

Slow-Cooked Lamb Chops with Oregano

Prep time: 15 min • **Cook time:** 2 hours • **Yield:** 2 servings

Ingredients	*Directions*
2 large lamb chops or steaks with bones (1 pound including bone), visible fat removed **Fine sea salt and fresh ground pepper to taste** **3 tablespoons fresh lemon juice** **1 teaspoon dried oregano** **1 bay leaf** **1 cup sliced onions** **½ cup white wine** **½ cup chicken broth** **Fresh chopped parsley, garnish**	*1* Place the lamb in a single layer in a 9-x-12-inch glass baking dish. Sprinkle salt and pepper over the meat and drizzle with lemon juice. Sprinkle the grated peel and oregano over the lamb and drizzle with olive oil. Place a bay leaf between the chops. Cover the dish with plastic wrap and refrigerate 4 hours or more. *2* Preheat the oven to 300°F. *3* Heat a skillet over high heat. Place the lamb in the skillet and brown on both sides before placing it back into the baking dish. Sprinkle the onions over the meat and pour in the wine and broth. *4* Cover the dish with foil and cook for 2 or more hours until the meat is very tender. Serve hot with the parsley garnish. Don't eat any of the remaining fat.

Per serving: Calories 286; Total fat: 14g; Saturated fat: 5g; Cholesterol: 102mg; Sodium: 594mg; Carbohydrates: 8g; Fiber: 2g; Sugar: 3g; Protein: 30g.

Tip: Lamb chops are naturally fatty, so if any fat remains on the chop, discard the fat.

(Recipe by Annabel Cohen)

Part IV

Incorporating Lifestyle Practices for Success

Four advantages of taking a brisk walk

Walking is great exercise and a great way to clear your head. Brisk walking actually has numerous benefits, so make sure you include brisk walking in your exercise regimen and do it on a regular basis. A brisk walk

- ✔ **Burns fat:** Brisk walking is fueled nearly exclusively through fat metabolism, which is why it's an ideal form of exercise while fasting and after an intense workout — two activities that release fatty acids into the bloodstream.

- ✔ **Improves heart health:** It's no wonder that cultures that walk more, live longer.

- ✔ **Improves mood:** Brisk walking outdoors brings you closer to nature, releases endorphins, and promotes overall well-being.

- ✔ **Strengthens bones:** Brisk walking is a safe and gentle introduction back to exercise and quickly serves to strengthen the bones, joints, and muscles. Brisk walking, in fact, is for everyone.

Visit www.dummies.com/extras/fastdiets for additional information about incorporating fasting into your daily lifestyle.

In this part...

- Examine the science behind exercising in a fasted state and how it can help you burn more fat, build muscle, and rejuvenate cells more effectively and efficiently than exercising in a non-fasted state.

- Find out how much and how frequently you should be exercising while fasting and how the two combined states can improve your abilities to reach your goals.

- Understand the differences and benefits that different types of exercise (weight training, metabolic conditioning, and cardio) while in a fasted state have on your body.

- Try some different exercises, such as the kettlebell swing, the goblet squat, and the Turkish get-up, with detailed instructions about how to perform the exercises safely and effectively in order to help you blast fat, build strength, and increase mobility.

- Grasp how stress affects both your body and mind, as well as how you can mitigate stress and anxiety in order to live your healthiest life.

- Discover techniques that can help you improve your sleep capacity and help you establish a natural rhythm akin to what your ancestors had.

Chapter 11

Comprehending the Effects of Fasting on Exercise and Vice Versa

In This Chapter

▶ Understanding the restorative power of fasting and exercise

▶ Using exercise and fasting to burn fat

▶ Getting leaner and building muscle

Exercise and fasting go together. They increase the effects of each other. In other words, exercise makes fasting better.

You can also say that fasting makes exercise better, because the relationship is reciprocal. One feeds the other, so to speak, and it doesn't matter which angle you approach it from. Whether you add exercise to fasting, or fasting to exercise, the net effect is the same.

This chapter covers how fasting can affect exercise and how exercise can affect fasting. The combination of fasting and exercise burns more fat than either one conducted independently. Furthermore, we discuss how fasting makes it easier for you to put on lean muscle mass, if that is a priority of yours (and it should be your priority).

 Ease into any fasted exercise, especially if you're beginning an exercise program for the first time, if you haven't exercised in a long time, or especially if you're a newbie with fasting. Although fasted exercise is one of the most natural and beneficial things for your body, it's a *stressor*. (It places a demand upon the body, which over time forces an adaptation. This is why it works.) As a result, enter into it carefully.

We do recommend that you enter into one at a time, which means if you've never fasted before and have been out of the business of intense exercise for quite some time, then acclimate yourself to fasting and exercise separately before combining the two.

The Lowdown on Fasting and Exercising: Why They Provide the Best Results

Combining fasting and exercise is the single most powerful decision you can make. In fact, being in a fasted state and exercising does more to restore the body to vibrant health than any cleanse, detox, or any other bogus supplement regimen could ever hope to do.

Almost all conventional wisdom on fasting and exercise is preposterously untrue. Many food companies would writhe in great pain if fasting were to ever be widely embraced. Cereal companies, in particular, would suffer (as they should!) to repay the karmic debt for propagating the idiotic idea that "breakfast is the most important meal of the deal" — the motto that serves only to keep their wallets full and your stomach fat.

If you have the choice either to exercise fasted or to exercise fed, the better option is to exercise fasted. Exercising fed offers virtually no benefits that you can't get from exercising fasted. On the other hand, exercising fasted has numerous benefits that you can't get from exercising fed.

In these sections, we cover the ins and outs of exercising fasted and reveal the truth that the two together can bring about the results that you want.

Understanding the link between the two

Fasting and exercise are forms of hardship, and the principle in physiology states that the body will adapt to certain hardships to maintain a state of equilibrium. The hardships of fasting and exercise, however, not only permit the body to adapt, but to thrive.

What we mean by this is that the adaptation benefits of these hardships are enormous — as long as those hardships are applied in a reasonable manner. Meaning, the body will get leaner, grow stronger, detoxify itself, and even regenerate itself when under such stresses.

Now what's truly remarkable about fasting and exercise is that when the two hardships are combined, they increase the positive effects of each other. For example, you would expect there to be a fat-burning benefit to be had from both fasting and intense exercise, and you would be right, but when you combine the two, you experience an even more profound fat-burning effect.

In short, you can expect any single benefit of either fasting or exercise to be increased when you combine the two hardships, such as:

- ✔ Fat loss (in scientific terms, *increased lipolysis*)
- ✔ Increased lean muscle tissue (improved mTOR sensitivity)
- ✔ Improved insulin sensitivity
- ✔ Cellular cleansing and detoxification
- ✔ Increased natural growth hormone

Refer to Chapter 2 for more discussion about these benefits and what happens in your body.

Determining your energy level

You may expect that exercising while fasted will result in less energy. Some people may experience lower energy levels, but it's only temporary. Over time the body adapts to fasted exercise and begins to pull energy more efficiently from stores in the body — such as fat and carbohydrate stores — rather than relying on a continuous sugar stream to fuel intense bouts of exercise. This process typically takes no longer than two weeks.

With fasting, you'll have a more continuous stream of energy for workouts — no more sugar crashes or burnouts — just clean, sustainable energy. In order to do so, you also need to eat well when you're not fasting, which means eating a diet rich in quality meats and seafood, healthy fats, fresh vegetables, and some fruits.

Be patient and give your body time to adapt to the changes of working out in a fasted state. In other words, don't judge fasted exercise by the first workout; stick it out for at least two weeks before passing any judgments.

Chapter 2 discusses how fasting serves to increase adrenal response, which also provides for additional energy while working out (as well as an increase in fat burning).

Avoiding food before a workout

To maximize the benefits of fasting and exercise together, you should eat nothing before a workout. The best way to make this work, of course, is to exercise in the morning hours before your first meal. For most of the fasting protocols outlined in this book, the best time to work out is before noon. Doing so allows you to break your fast immediately after your workout, which is yet another ideal situation, because the food from that meal will go almost exclusively toward feeding and repairing hungry muscle tissue, rather than shuttling into fat cells.

If you can't make morning exercise a part of your routine, then at least refrain from eating for at least two to three hours before you work out.

If you're prone to dizzy spells or anything of that sort while working out, we suggest that you ease yourself into working out in a fully fasted state. Consider doing the following:

1. **Eliminate all sugar from your diet — except the sugars that come naturally from fruits and vegetables.**

   Doing so can help to ensure a more stable blood sugar throughout training sessions.

2. **Eat mostly lean proteins and healthy fats before a workout, limiting carbohydrate intake.**

3. **After you're comfortable with the first two steps, start to push your pre-workout meal further and further back.**

   Take your time and progress at a comfortable pace.

You can also take branched chain amino acids to provide fuel before and after exercise. *Amino acids* are the building blocks of protein, and the *branched chain* amino acids, which are leucine, isoleucine, and valine, are essential amino acids, meaning humans must acquire them through diet, because the human body is unable to produce them on its own. What's neat about branched chain amino acids, however, is that they're metabolized directly in muscle tissue (rather than in the liver where most other amino acids are metabolized), which means they serve as a nearly immediate fuel source for muscle tissue. They also help to prevent muscle breakdown from intense exercise. Supplementing with branched chain amino acids before and after training may be a useful strategy if you wish to add muscle mass. They're also a good alternative for people who have sensitivity issues to whey protein because of lactose intolerance or other related issues.

Knowing what to eat (and whether you should) after exercise

Post-workout nutrition is essential. Your muscles are desperately hungry for nutrients in a specific time-frame after your exercise. As a general rule, you should wait 30 minutes after your intense workout sessions before you ingest anything. This time gives your body a chance to discover how to handle the stresses of exercise on its own (rather than always relying on the use of dietary supplementation), as it naturally increases antioxidant production to combat and reverse oxidative damage sustained through intense exercise. In turn, this strengthens your own natural antioxidant system.

This period also prolongs the amount of time your body will continue to burn off stored body fat. As soon as you eat post workout — particularly if you eat a carbohydrate-rich diet — you begin to shut off the fat-burning processes set forth by fasting and exercise. We recommend that you use this 30-minute waiting period to perform some low-intensity cardiovascular activity, such as hiking or brisk walking. Don't just sit around and do nothing. Make sure you move.

After 30 minutes, make sure you consume a post-workout meal, which should be your largest of the day to give the muscles the materials they need to repair themselves. You can cram in a considerable amount of calories post workout (even carbohydrates) and not have to worry about any of it being stored as fat. Even if you aren't all that hungry, be sure to at least consume some protein 30 to 60 minutes post workout.

In this meal, include a high-quality protein source, because protein provides the building blocks for muscle (amino acids). Meat, poultry, and seafood are all great options. And if you're going to have some starchy carbohydrates, such as a sweet potato, post workout is the time to have it, because it will go directly toward replenishing muscle and liver *glycogen* (the stored carbo-hydrates) that are heavily depleted through intense exercise. For example, a perfect post-workout meal can include salmon, asparagus, and a sweet potato.

To control insulin and manage hunger, eat your food in a specific order. Start with the most nutrient-dense and fibrous vegetables (like a green salad). Then move to proteins and healthy fats (like salmon). Finally, move onto the denser, starchy carb sources (like sweet potatoes).

If whole foods aren't an option for you post workout, then you may consider supplementation, such as branched chain amino acids or whey protein. Whey protein, so long as it comes from grass-fed cows and doesn't contain any oils or artificial sweeteners, is a powerful muscle builder.

Fasting and Exercise = More Fat Burning

Fasted exercise is the most potent fat burner on the planet. More potent than any diet pill, we assure you, safer too, and much more economical. If you want to lose weight more effectively, then combining fasting with exercise will satisfy you. To burn fat and ultimately lose weight, combine high-intensity exercise (such as heavy weightlifting and metabolic conditioning) with low-intensity exercise (such as walking and hiking), in that order while in a fasted state.

The reasoning is simple. High-intensity exercise, primarily fueled by carbohydrates and not fat, serves the useful purpose of releasing fatty acids into the bloodstream, where they can then be *oxidized* (burned off). This releasing of fatty acids is in large part due to the adrenaline response you receive from high-intensity bouts of exercise. Sprinting is a good example.

After you complete your high intensity workout session, which should typically last no longer than 30 minutes, you should immediately enter into a form of low intensity exercise. Downshifting from high intensity to low intensity allows your body to continue to burn the aforementioned fatty acids, because fat, not carbs, fuels low intensity aerobic activity.

This biological trickery, if you can call it that, is all you need. It doesn't need to be complicated. For example, 20 minutes of sprints followed by 30 to 40 minutes of brisk walking is effective for hacking fat right off the body — of course if it's done while in a fasted state.

If you're looking for something that is a little lower impact, you can perform kettlebell swings, on and off, for 20 minutes. Try 15 seconds on, 15 seconds off, doing as many swings in each 15-second working block as you can with good form. It's brutal, but effective. Be sure to follow with a brisk walk as well.

To further assist you, here is a brief list of our favorite high-intensity movements. (We discuss them in Chapter 12.)

- Dead lifts
- Goblet squats
- Kettlebell swings
- Pull-ups
- Push-ups
- Sprinting
- Turkish get-ups

Intensity isn't necessarily related to how much you sweat. Perceived exertion is one measure of intensity, for sure, but you should also consider other forms. The amount of weight you lift is also a form of intensity. More weight means more intensity. So, although lifting a heavy load for one to three reps at a time probably won't leave you huffing or puffing, it still counts as a form of intense exercise, because it still imparts a large amount of stress on the system.

After you do your high-intensity exercise, you'll want to do a low-intensity activity (for between 30 to 60 minutes) to help the fat-burning process. Here is a brief list of our favorite low-intensity activities:

- Biking/cycling
- Engaging in most recreational sports
- Hiking
- Playing Frisbee
- Swimming
- Walking

Don't go too hard with these low-intensity activities or else they won't be low intensity anymore. Remember, lightly keep on the move, have some fun, and let loose a little bit. At any given time you should be able to talk during these low-intensity activities, because it gives you a good idea that you're keeping it at the right intensity. If you're too winded to speak, then ease up a bit.

Building More Lean Muscle

Fasted exercise won't build you more muscle, but it will make it possible to add lean muscle mass more efficiently. In other words, through fasting (which improves insulin sensitivity), and by being leaner (which means you typically have improved insulin sensitivity than someone who is overweight and/or insulin resistant), you have the ability to utilize nutrients more efficiently, specifically protein. Fasting basically helps to reset the mechanisms behind protein *synthesis,* which is the biological process of muscle building and rejuvenation, allowing you to potentially build more lean muscle with fewer available nutrients.

The human body has a mechanism known as the mammalian target of rapamycin, or mTOR for short, which is the body's primary muscle-building gene. Fasting primes the muscle-building machinery by increasing insulin sensitivity and suppressing mTOR. You can almost think of mTOR as a spring. When it's suppressed, it gains potential and the more it is suppressed, the more potential it gains. When mTOR is unleashed, it does its job much more powerfully. Refer to Chapter 2 for more information about the science of fasting and the role of insulin and mTOR.

You can also hack into your hormonal hardwiring and jump-start the muscle-building process with intense exercise. When you suppress mTOR, you increase the potential for efficiently building lean muscle.

When you combine fasting with intense exercise, you can imagine the types of muscle-building results you can expect. So, in simple terms, if you fast through the morning hours, lift hard and heavy for 30 to 40 minutes, and then consume your largest meal as your post-workout meal about 30 to 60 minutes after your intense workout, you can bet that just about all of that meal is going to go directly to building lean, dense muscle tissue.

If you're following the micro-fasting protocol (which is perhaps the most convenient protocol; refer to Chapter 6), then the best time to train is the late morning or early afternoon hours, so that when you finish your workout, you may go directly into breaking your fast. The same goes for the Warrior Diet as we discuss in Chapter 7.

Sprinting, because it is a form of intense exercise, is a perfect way to activate your muscle-building genes while fasted. So, when in doubt, sprint! Sprinting is fun, primal, and effective. It boosts natural growth hormone, scorches body fat, and strengthens the heart muscle in a way that no other form of exercise can.

If you're following the 5:2 Diet (see Chapter 5), then the best approach is to either work out first thing in the morning before you break your fast or cram as much time in between your breakfast and workout session as possible.

If you're following intermittent fasting (refer to Chapter 4), then try to time your workout around the end of your fasting period, as you would if you were micro-fasting. The difference, though, is that your workout may fall at any hour, depending on when you started your fasting period.

Time your most intensive bouts of exercise in such a manner that you may resume eating upon the completion of your workout and work in micro-bouts of exercise throughout your fasting period. These small bursts of exercise work to boost the positive effects of fasting. For example, a short bout of sprints, two minutes of kettlebell swings, or even a set or two of pull-ups are all fine examples of exercises you can do to get better results in building lean muscle.

Restoring the Body

We're sorry to say but there are no easy solutions to health and fitness. There are only proven strategies, all of which, without exception, include a form of hardship. Fasting and intense exercise combined are the two choicest examples — the finest hardships nature has to offer. Don't shun the two. Embrace them together.

These sections delve into how exercise and fasting together can restore the body. The science, by the way, only serves to prove what humans have known to be true all along — that fasting, especially when combined with intense exercise, is very good for you.

Cleaning out the system

Fasting triggers a nearly miraculous cleansing process throughout the entire body. It not only permits organs and glands a much-needed rest, particularly the digestive system, but it also allows for the body's natural home-cleaning mechanisms (including white blood cells, enzymes, and so on) to course through your body and take out the trash. That trash includes anything from damaged cells, metabolic waste, toxins, pollutants, unwelcome bacteria or microbes, and even impacted feces.

Muscle tissue enters into a restoration process as well, as old, damaged tissue is recycled when you enter into a fast. This process keeps muscles healthy, young, and strong.

To be clear, unless you live in an immaculately clean vacuum, which is clearly impossible even if such a space existed, you're bound to accumulate waste, toxins, and pollutants over time through your diet and exposure to less-than-ideal environmental conditions, and the only way to purge these from your body is to fast.

Adding exercise into the mix accelerates this natural process of cleaning and purging. In fact, it actually supercharges it, so to speak. Specifically, it boosts the rate at which your body will recycle dirty, damaged cells and kick starts the process of building new muscle tissue.

If you don't purge your system from time to time through fasting and exercise, your body will find less effective and less desirable ways to clean itself out for you, such as acne or diarrhea. In fact, foul body odor, putrid breath, pimples, runny stool, and other undesirables are all indicators that your body is overrun by toxins and is in desperate need of a cleanse.

What's more, the more toxins you accumulate and the less time you take to purge those toxins, the greater the risk of your body just "giving up" and succumbing to any number of fatal conditions, certainly not limited to, but including cancer.

Feeling lightheaded, nauseous, or any unpleasantness while fasting and exercise isn't the result of a nutritional deficiency. These symptoms referred to as a *healing crisis,* which is a natural and admittedly annoying period of withdrawal as your body rids itself of toxins, similar to a hangover. They aren't a sign to stop fasting and exercising, but rather a sign that what you're doing is working.

Impacting the brain in a positive manner

Your brain also needs cleansing because it hoards trash just like any other organ. In the brain, this trash is largely an accumulation of damaged cells and other assorted toxins. Fasting specifically acts to stimulate *autophagy,* which is the process through which the brain cleans itself. More specifically it's when the cells purge waste material and repair themselves. It's an amazing rejuvenation process, to be sure, and absolutely essential for overall brain health and longevity.

The brain needs to be stressed and stimulated like any other organ in order to stay healthy, and the best way to positively impact the brain is through fasting and exercise.

A lack of this cleansing process may lead to any number of neurological diseases including Alzheimer's disease and dementia. Insufficient cleansing of the brain also leads to *neurodegeneration,* a fancy term to describe a state where the brain doesn't function or develop properly. Fasting has proven to increase autophagy and restore vitality to the brain. (Interestingly, fasting has long been used overseas as a successful treatment for many psychological disorders such as neurosis. In Russia, they call fasting "the hunger cure.") Together, fasting and exercise increase autophagy even more. In fact, the combination of fasting and intense exercise is the most therapeutic remedy for the body and the mind, as well as perhaps the most potent preventive measure you can take against the onset of any neurological diseases.

The science also shows that fasting and exercise boost *neurogenesis,* which is the growth of new brain cells. Fasting and exercise also strengthen the brain's synaptic infrastructure, or the lines of communication between neurons. This means better, healthier brain function all around.

Chapter 12

Putting Together Your Fasting Exercise Program

To get the most out of fasting, exercise is imperative. Although any exercise at all is better than none, certainly some forms of exercise are more effective than others — especially when you want to boost the positive effects of fasting, such as burning more fat, building more muscle, and forging healthier cells.

You can't realize vitality without a delicate interplay between fasting and exercise. Fasting alone is enough to restore some vigor to the body, no doubt, and so is exercise alone, but when you can combine the two, and do so in a balanced, healthy manner, you amplify the benefits of both dramatically.

This chapter helps you to construct your exercise program. We discuss the three key components — heavy lifting, metabolic training, and light aerobic activity — to a successful exercise program. As we explain how you can incorporate these components into your exercise program, we walk you through some of them step by step, and provide plenty of photos to show you how to do the different exercises.

Boosting Strength and Building Muscle with Resistance Training: The How-To

If you want to get stronger, the only way to do so is to move against resistance. We use the term "resistance," and not the term "weights," because resistance doesn't have to be external. *Resistance* simply is the opposition to some type of force. For example, a push-up, for many, is a challenging resistance exercise that requires no external equipment. If you're advanced in your exercise routine and the push-up movement is easy for you, and you want to increase the resistance, then you can try a one-arm push-up, or a one-arm, one-leg push-up. We simply want to demonstrate that weight training isn't the only form of resistance training. You don't need to lift weights to get strong.

Strength is a function of generating tension in the muscles. The harder you can tense your muscles, the more force (strength) you can exert. Strength is a habit. It's a skill that anyone can develop over time. All you need to do is practice, practice, and more practice. If you can understand that strength is a high and delicate art and not a sort of random nonsense as most people treat it, you'll have the ability to acquire strength beyond what you probably ever thought possible.

Debunking the conventional wisdom about strength

Some people have misconceptions about what it really means to be strong. You don't need big muscles to be strong. That is, and always will be, a false claim. The ability to generate tension in your muscles isn't related to muscle size, but rather, the efficiency of your nervous system. The central nervous system (which you can think of as your control center or operations manager) dictates how hard you can tense your muscles.

The more you practice moving against resistance, the more tension your central nervous system allows. The body naturally seeks efficiency and will adapt to physiological demands placed upon it (which is known as the *law of* *adaptation* to imposed demands). As long as you continue to move against resistance, your central nervous system will aim to increase the efficiency of that movement. It does so in large part by allowing for more tension in the muscles.

Take for example, the gymnast, who may be, pound for pound, the strongest athlete in the world. The classic gymnastic physique isn't overly muscular, certainly not bulky, yet a gymnast can display nearly superhuman levels of strength. Why? Well, the gymnast has a finely tuned nervous system, which means the gymnast's movement is efficient. The gymnast has learned the skill of strength, so to speak. And that's all strength really is, a skill.

These sections explain how you can practice strength, including when you can exercise and what the types of exercises you can do to help you develop strength.

Determining when and how much

If you wanted to get good at the piano, a good teacher would tell you to practice every day. So then, if you want to get strong, isn't it a good idea to practice strength every day?

Well, yes and no. Unlike piano playing, strength training takes a much heavier toll on the body, and your body needs time to recover because through the processes of recovery your body adapts and gets stronger. Although there are ways to practice strength every day and still recover from it, we're going to give you a more reasonable approach and prescribe three to four days a week of strength training.

The strength-training schedule that we recommend is as follows:

On/on/off/on/on/off/off

That's two days of strength training followed by a day of rest, and then two more days of strength training followed by two more days of rest. You can fit it into your week however your schedule allows. For example, the most classic approach puts your strength training on Monday, Tuesday, Thursday, and Friday, with the weekend open. If you work weekends and have Tuesday and Wednesday off, you can revise the schedule so that you work out Thursday, Friday, Sunday, and Monday with Saturday Tuesday, and Wednesday off.

You can get away with less if you simply don't have the time in your schedule. Although we believe four days a week is ideal, you can still have great results if you strength train only two to three days a week. Remember, some is always better than none.

As for how much, we recommend that in any given strength-training session, you train only two to three full-body exercises, which we walk you through in the later "Knowing which exercises to do" section.

As for how to go about your strength training, you can take three general approaches, all of which are effective:

Practice sets

You can practice sets for time rather than a predetermined amount of sets or reps. A *set* comprises of repetitions (often called *reps*). A *repetition* is how many times you perform an exercise in a row. So, for example, two sets of five reps of the squat means you perform five repetitions of the squat, rest for whatever time deemed necessary, and then perform another five repetitions of the squat.

When working practice sets, you put a certain amount of time on the clock. We recommend 20 to 30 minutes. From there, you just practice whatever exercise you may have on the menu that day. When practicing a movement, keep the repetitions low (less than five) and rest as long as you need between sets.

Practice sets are about accumulating as many quality repetitions as possible in the allotted time. The key word is *quality*. Again, rest as long as you need, but as little as you have to between the sets to execute the exercise with impeccably good form.

For example, say you want to work a practice set with the push-up. You put 20 to 30 minutes on the clock, and practice sets of the push-up. You can practice sets of one, two, three, four, or five, but don't go any higher than five, because fatigue will start to set in and compromise your movement quality. If say you choose to do practice sets of three reps, you do three push-ups, rest for a short bit, do another set of three push-ups, rest, and so on for the full 20 to 30 minutes. As time wears off the clock, you'll get more tired and may need more time between sets. Just make sure you don't allow your fatigue to affect your form. Take slightly longer rests between the sets if you need. You can even practice ladders (see the next section).

Be sure to keep track of your repetitions, because the next time you do the practice set, your goal should be to beat your previous record.

Ladders

Ladders are ascending sets comprised of rungs. A *rung* is simply the term used for sets in a ladder. If a ladder has three rungs, then it consists of three sets. If it has five rungs, it consists of five sets. Each rung, however, typically consists of different reps, because the sets in a ladder ascend. For example, if you do a set of one squat, then a set of two, then a set of three, you have just performed a three-rung ladder.

For strength training, the best practices are

✔ Three-rung ladders, such as 1, 2, 3 (one rep, followed by two reps, followed by three reps)

✔ Five-rung ladders, such as 1, 2, 3, 4, 5 (one rep, followed by two reps, followed by three reps, followed by four reps, followed by five reps)

For most exercises, performing two, three-rung or two, five-rung ladders is plenty, especially if you're going heavy with the lift, which you should be.

To paint a clearer picture, say your strength training day calls for two, three-rung ladders of pull-ups. You do the following:

1. **Perform one pull-up.**

2. **Rest for as long as you need.**

3. **Perform two pull-ups.**

4. **Rest again.**

5. **When you're ready, perform three pull-ups.**

6. **Start back at one pull-up and work your way through Steps 1 to 5.**

Three-by-three or five-by-five

Three sets of three (3 x 3) or five sets of five (5 x 5) are also classic strength-training protocols. They're also the easiest to understand. Three sets of three means that you perform three repetitions of any given exercise three times. For example, if you're to work 3 x 3 on the dead lift, then you perform three dead lifts, rest for as long as necessary, three dead lifts again, rest for as long as necessary, and finally, three more dead lifts. The same goes for 5 x 5.

Knowing which exercises to do

When beginning an exercise program, the best exercises are the biggest exercises — squats, dead lifts, push-ups, pull-ups, lunges, kettlebell swings, and hanging leg raises, to name just a few. These full body movements work the most muscle groups at one time (unlike many single joint type of movements, such as bicep curls or tricep extensions), and, in turn, offer the highest calorie burn and strength returns.

We don't have enough room in this book to cover all the exercises that we suggest you do, so we focus on six of our favorite beginner strength-building movements. When you're ready for a more in-depth explanation of exercises, look in our book *Paleo Workouts For Dummies* (John Wiley & Sons, Inc.).

These sections focus on the following six exercises to help you get started with your strength-training program:

✔ Dead lift

✔ Goblet squat

✔ Push-up

✔ Pull-up

✔ Turkish get-up

✔ Kettlebell swing

Dead lift

The *dead lift* is how you pick things up off the ground, or how you *should* pick things up off the ground. The dead lift is basically a hip hinge, meaning you initiate the movement by pushing back your butt and hinging at the hips.

The dead lift strengthens the *entire posterior chain* (in plain English your backside), which consists primarily of your hamstrings, your butt, and your lower back. The dead lift is a monstrous strength-building movement, because when done properly, it allows you to move a very large amount of weight, especially when done with a barbell. But starting out, we show you how to perform it with a kettlebell, which makes the movement a bit more accessible for beginners. We don't recommend moving onto the barbell, and really loading up the weight, until your kettlebell dead lift is near perfected.

Here is how to do the dead lift:

1. **Stand over the kettlebell with a shoulder-width stance and point your toes slightly out as Figure 12-1 shows.**

   Take your time and ensure that you begin the movement with proper posture. Think, "long, tall spine."

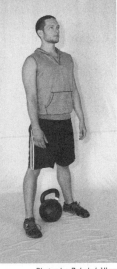

Figure 12-1:
Be sure the kettlebell is positioned between your feet, not in front of them.

Photos by: Rebekah Ulmer

2. **Push your butt back as if you're reaching for a bench that's just out of reach, and continue to push your butt back as far as you possibly can without falling over backward.**

Your knees will bend, but they shouldn't come forward. Be sure to keep your back flat at all times (see Figure 12-2). There should be a straight line from the back of your head down through your tailbone. Dead lifting with a rounded back is an unsafe and weak position.

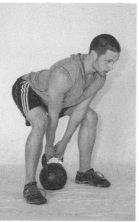

Figure 12-2:
Keep your back flat at all times.

Photos by: Rebekah Ulmer

3. **After your butt is as far back as it will go, reach down and grab hold of the kettlebell.**

4. **Take a deep breath into your belly, push your heels hard into the ground, and stand straight up to finish the movement.**

Don't lean back at the top of the dead lift; just stand tall as Figure 12-3 shows. Keep your butt and abs tight.

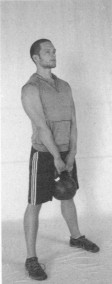

Figure 12-3:
Be sure to
extend your
hips and
knees fully
at the top.

Photos by: Rebekah Ulmer

5. **Put the weight down exactly the way you picked it up.**

Goblet squat

The goblet squat, a movement invented by renowned strength coach Dan John, is perhaps the most simplistic, but effective squat variation in existence.

What's great about the goblet squat is that it's almost impossible to do wrong, making it a perfect beginner squatting variation. Just because it's easy and great for beginners, however, doesn't mean that it's of no use to veterans. The goblet squat allows for *heavy loading* (it makes the movement more difficult, which means you just pick up a heavier weight), just like front squats (which is essentially the same movement, but done with a barbell instead of kettlebells or dumbbells), so after you're comfortable with the movement, you can start to go heavy with it.

Follow these steps to do the goblet squat:

1. **Grab a kettlebell or a dumbbell and hold it snuggly in front of your chest.**

   This is called the *goblet position*.

2. **Assume a shoulder-width stance — maybe a smidgen wider — and point your toes slightly out (refer to Figure 12-4).**

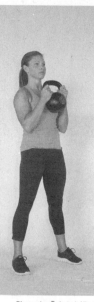

Figure 12-4:
The weight
also acts
as a coun-
terbalance
to help you
achieve
more depth.

Photos by: Rebekah Ulmer

3. **Pull yourself down between your legs and go as low as you can with a flat back while keeping your heels on the ground.**

Imagine you're trying to sit down on a curb. Don't forget to breathe. Take a deep breath into your belly before you lower into the squat, and breathe forcefully out as you ascend (refer to Figure 12-5).

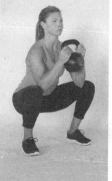

Figure 12-5:
Breathe
deeply
before low-
ering into
the squat.

Photos by: Rebekah Ulmer

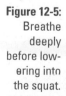

4. **After you hit your maximum depth, push your heels into the ground, and stand straight up to finish the movement.**

    Your hips and shoulders should ascend at the same rate, not one before the other.

Push-up

The push-up is the classic gym class exercise that most people do incorrectly. Here, we're going to make sure you do it correctly. The push-up is still really one of the best, if not the best, upper-body strength-building exercises you can do. It hits the chest, the shoulders, the triceps, the abs, and a few other things here and there.

We realize that push-ups by themselves aren't all that difficult for some people. But who said you need to limit yourself to only standard push-ups? After you're able to bang out 15 reps or more of the push-up, you can start the one-arm push-up, or the one-arm, one-leg push-up (both of which we discuss in *Paleo Workouts For Dummies*).

Here is how you can to do a perfect push-up:

1. **Lie flat on your stomach, face down, with your arms by your sides (as in Figure 12-6).**

2. **Lift your arms back up behind you as high as you can, but keep your elbows straight.**

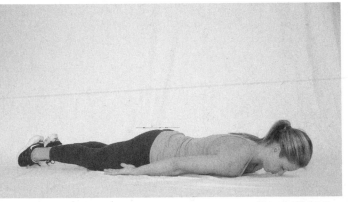

Figure 12-6: Set up your push-up from the bottom, like this, to ensure a foolproof setup.

Photos by: Rebekah Ulmer

3. **Bend your elbows 90 degrees and plant your hands on the ground.**

    They should fall almost directly in line with your sternum. At this point, your arms should be tucked in closely to your sides, your elbows bent at about 90 degrees, and your forearms perpendicular to the ground (refer to Figure 12-7).

If you've never done a push-up like this, it will likely feel more difficult at first, but keep your elbows in close to your body. In the long run, you'll be stronger.

Figure 12-7: Notice that the forearms are vertical. This is what makes for a good starting position.

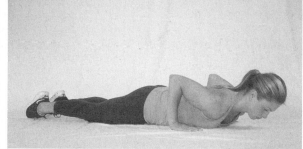

Photos by: Rebekah Ulmer

4. **Tuck in your toes, tense your whole body, and push yourself up to the top of a push-up position (see Figure 12-8).**

Your chest, stomach, and hips all rise and descend at the same rate. In other words, when done right, your body should ascend and descend as a stiff and single unit — a plank of wood — and not in a wavelike or wormlike manner.

Figure 12-8: Keep your back straight at all times during a push-up.

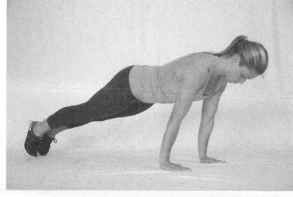

Photos by: Rebekah Ulmer

5. **Lower yourself back down, keeping your elbows in tight, and repeat the movement.**

Pull-up

The pull-up is also a classic upper-body strength builder and the perfect complement to the push-up, because when you push, you must also pull. Although a pull-up is more difficult, you can do one. Even if you can't right now, with some practice, you can do one.

Here's how to do a proper pull-up:

1. **Hang from a bar or a set of rings with a shoulder-width grip as Figure 12-9 shows.**

   Make sure your palms are facing away from you for a pull-up. If they're facing toward you, then you're doing a chin-up.

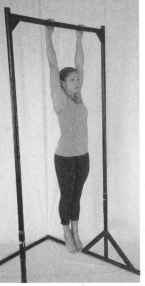

Figure 12-9: Make sure you start in a full dead hang with your elbows fully extended.

Photos by: Rebekah Ulmer

2. **Tighten your whole body by squeezing your butt, bracing your abs, sucking down your shoulders, and bringing your body into a hanging plank position (refer to Figure 12-10).**

   Try to create as much space between your shoulders and ears as possible. A *hanging plank position,* also known as the *hollow position,* is a straight line from the back of your head down through your tailbone. Just holding the hanging plank position can help tremendously to build the strength needed for a full pull-up.

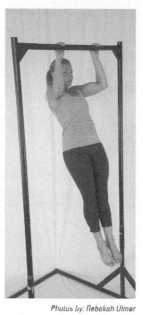

Figure 12-10:
Get your
body into
a hanging
plank posi-
tion for a
proper pull-
up.

Photos by: Rebekah Ulmer

3. **Pull up by driving your elbows down hard toward your hips (as in Figure 12-11).**

   Don't use any momentum or sway when performing pull-ups. Focus on getting stronger. Try to get your throat against the bar. An even better finish is to get your chest against the bar.

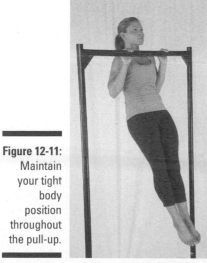

Figure 12-11:
Maintain
your tight
body
position
throughout
the pull-up.

Photos by: Rebekah Ulmer

4. **Descend under control and back to a full dead hang position with your elbows fully extended.**

   Half-reps don't count.

Turkish get-up

The Turkish get-up is one of the most comprehensive, compound movements in existence today, because it has you moving just about every joint in your body. The purpose of this exercise is to get up off the ground while supporting a weight overhead.

This movement simultaneously works elements of *mobility* (the ability to move through a range of motion) and *stability* (the ability to resist changes in joint position) in the shoulders, hips, and core. It's also a marvelous strength builder, when you're ready to go heavy with it. The Turkish get-up, or get-up for short, forges resilient shoulders, supple hips, and a bulletproof midsection.

Here's how you can do the Turkish get-up:

1. **Lie on your back in the prone position.**

   Fully extend your arms and legs and angle them away from your body at roughly 45 degrees. Your right arm should run parallel to your right leg and vice versa. It should sort of look like the bottom of a snow angel position.

2. **To work on your right side, directly press your right arm in line with your sternum (mid-chest) as if you were performing a one-arm bench press (this is also the arm that will be holding the weight).**

   Don't perform this movement with any weight until you have each of these steps mastered. Bend your right knee and plant your right heel relatively close to your butt.

   Your right heel should be relatively close to your butt, not directly. Take as much time as you need to set up correctly (as Figure 12-12 shows). (If you're working on the left side, you should do the opposite with the setup and the following directions.)

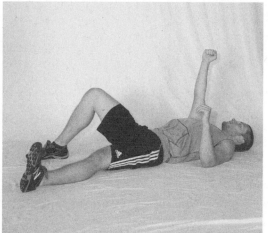

Figure 12-12:
A proper setup is crucial to execute the Turkish get-up.

Photos by: Rebekah Ulmer

3. **To execute the roll, push hard into your right-planted heel, pull hard from your left-planted elbow, drive your chest upward, and prop yourself up onto your left forearm.**

The roll is perhaps the most difficult portion of the get-up and perhaps the most beneficial as well. Rolling up off the ground is an essential movement skill that people tend to lose as they age (because of a severe lack of practice), but it serves the useful function of knitting together your core.

This movement is a roll, not a crunch or a sit-up. Lead with a proud chest, and keep your back flat. Keep your right arm extended straight overhead. (Imagine you're balancing a half cup of water on your fist at all times; don't let it spill!) If you lead this movement with your head and round your back, then you're doing it wrong. Check out Figure 12-13 for how it looks.

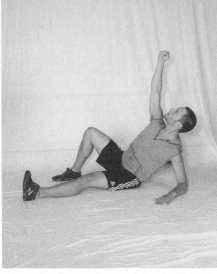

Figure 12-13:
Make sure
this part is
a roll, not
a crunch
or a sit-
up. When
rolling,
the spine
shouldn't
flex (bend).

Photos by: Rebekah Ulmer

4. **Move from your forearm up to your hand, by extending the elbow as in Figure 12-14.**

   However, don't lift your hand, instead, simply pivot on it. Don't let your shoulders shrug up in this position. Think about keeping as much distance between your shoulders and ears as possible. An effective, but somewhat crude cue that seems to do the trick is to pretend you're squishing a beetle.

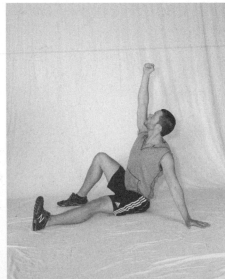

Figure 12-14:
Lock your
elbow fully
and turn
your fingers
back behind
you.

Photos by: Rebekah Ulmer

5. **Bridge by pushing your heel into the ground, squeezing your butt, and driving your hips up into the air.**

   You should be able to freely lift your straight leg off the ground in the bridge position as in Figure 12-15. If you can't, shift your weight onto the heel of your bent leg. Try your very best to come into a full bridge, but don't overextend.

Figure 12-15:
Lift your straight leg off the ground in the bridge position.

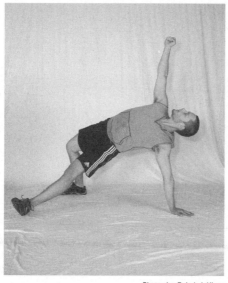

Photos by: Rebekah Ulmer

6. **Sweep your straight leg (in this case your left leg) back under your hips, planting your knee directly in line with your planted hand (refer to Figure 12-16).**

   When done correctly, your legs should form an "L" with one knee facing forward and the other knee facing outward. Don't try to sweep your leg back in such a manner that both knees face forward, like they would in a lunge position. This is awkward and will put you into a bad position.

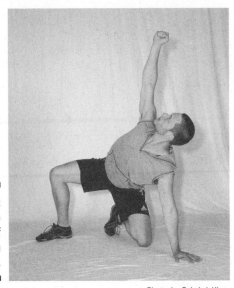

Photos by: Rebekah Ulmer

Figure 12-16:
The sweep
portion of
the Turkish
get-up.

7. **Simultaneously lift your planted hand and rotate your back leg to come up off the ground and into an overhead lunge position (refer to Figure 12-17).**

   In the starting position, firmly plant your back toes on the ground (not pointed behind you), so that you can push off your back leg just as much as your front leg to stand up.

   The movement of your back leg should look similar to a windshield wiper, as your back calf swings outward until both knees are pointed in the same direction.

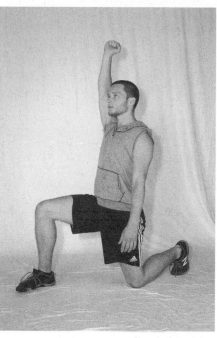

Figure 12-17:
After you reach this lunge position, look straight ahead.

Photos by: Rebekah Ulmer

8. To finish the Turkish get-up, stand up out of the lunge.

At the top of the Turkish get-up, there should be a straight line up through your legs, torso, and arm connecting the weight to the ground. Check out Figure 12-18.

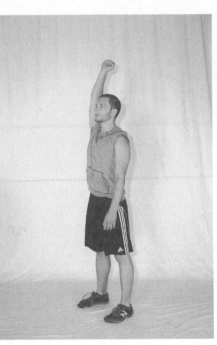

Figure 12-18:
The finish of
the Turkish
get-up.

Photos by: Rebekah Ulmer

You can reverse everything you just did — step-by-step — and return to the starting position.

Kettlebell swing

The kettlebell swing is simply the dead lift performed quickly and consecutively. It's an explosive hinging movement, where you swing a weight — in this case a kettlebell — between your legs, and then powerfully drive your hips forward to accelerate the bell upward.

The kettlebell swing helps to develop explosive power, similar to how a broad jump would, but without all the impact on the joints. Furthermore, high rep kettlebell swings melt fat like raw meat on a hot grill and are one of the best exercises for intense cardiovascular conditioning.

Here is how you can do the kettlebell swing:

1. **Stand a little bit behind a kettlebell (no more than a foot) with your feet shoulder width apart and your toes slightly out.**

2. **Hinge at the hips like you would for a dead lift, reach out, and grab the kettlebell (refer to Figure 12-19).**

In this position, you should look like a center about to hike back a foot-ball (the kettlebell).

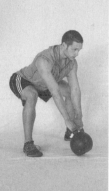

Figure 12-19: Always start with a flat back.

Photos by: Rebekah Ulmer

3. **Swing by hiking the kettlebell back between your legs as you would a football.**

   Be sure that your back remains flat at all times and that your shoulders don't dip below your knees as in Figure 12-20.

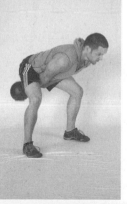

Figure 12-20: At the bottom of the kettlebell swing, you should look like a witch riding a broomstick.

Photos by: Rebekah Ulmer

4. **As soon as the kettlebell reaches the height of the backswing, explosively drive your hips forward and stand up as quickly as you can (refer to Figure 12-21).**

   Allow the kettlebell to float to about chest or eye level, but no higher. Also be sure to keep your butt tight and your belly tight at the top, so you don't overextend your hips or lean back at the top of the movement. Imagine that you're trying to jump, but don't let your heels leave the ground.

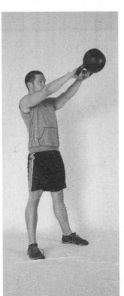

Figure 12-21:
The top of the kettle-bell swing.

Photos by: Rebekah Ulmer

5. **As soon as the kettlebell reaches about chest height, allow the downward motion to drop it back down into the backswing, and repeat the movement.**

   Don't try to control the downward motion of the kettlebell. Let gravity work. When the kettlebell reaches the low point, repeat the swing. Be sure that when you're done with your set of swings you set the kettlebell down safely, and with a flat back.

Putting it all together

Organizing your strength training doesn't need to be a confusing or overly complicated matter. To help you get started, in this section we provide you with a sample program where you can use the exercises that we discussed in the previous section.

Although you may want to design your own program, we encourage you to follow our plan for at least three months before you do so.

Tackling a few reminders

Before you start, here are a few additional considerations for you to remember:

- ✔ **For these lifts, use a weight that is between your five- and seven-rep maximum.** You shouldn't be able to lift the weight for more than five to seven consecutive repetitions. So, if you can't lift the weight at least five times, go lighter; if you can lift it for more than seven times, go heavier.

- ✔ **For the body weight exercises, such as push-ups and pull-ups, use the most difficult progression (or regression) that you can handle for five to seven repetitions.** For example, if a push-up is too easy for you, start to work toward a one-arm push-up. If a push-up is too difficult for you, start with a regression, such as performing a push-up with your hands elevated on a bench. The same goes for pull-ups; if they're too easy, start working toward the one-arm pull-up. If they're too difficult, start with *body weight rows* (do them with a set of exercise straps, where you lean back and pull yourself up from a more horizontal, rather than vertical position, making the movement somewhat easier), or *static holds* (holding yourself at the top of the pull-up bar for 3 to 5 seconds at a time and slowly lowering yourself down).

- ✔ **Don't increase the weight for three months.** The goal of this program is to start with a heavy load (a five- to seven-rep max) and to finish with that load feeling light(er). So, that means, for three months, leave the weight exactly where it is, even when it starts to feel light. After that happens, you can further refine your technique, and perform the lifts with more speed, power, and grace. After the initial three months, you may reevaluate your new five- to seven-rep max for all the lifts and then accordingly increase the weight. *Note:* The only exception to this rule is with kettlebell swings where you should use a weight that you can swing between 10 and 20 times.

- ✔ **Add metabolic conditioning on two to three days per week.** See the next section for more details. You should always perform metabolic training after your strength-training sessions and never before. If necessary, do them on separate days.

- ✔ **Never do more than you're comfortable doing.** Go at your own pace, but work diligently. Strength will come with practice. Use common sense and good judgment. If something feels unsafe, it probably is. Make sure you seek out a good coach and get your technique refined if necessary. Feel free to email me at patflynn@chroniclesofstrength.com, and I'll be happy to help you with your technique.

Looking at a sample week's workout

We suggest you stick to a schedule where you work out two days in a row, take one day off, work out two more days, and then take two days off. Here we spell out our workout plan for you to follow. We start our plan on a Monday, but if you need to begin on another day, that's fine. Just make sure you then stick to the schedule over the next seven days. Please refer to the earlier sections, "Determining when and how much" and "Knowing which exercises to do" for specifics.

Monday

Dead lift practice set: 20 to 30 minutes (use between 1–5 reps per set)

Turkish get-up ladder: 1, 2, 3, 1, 2, 3 (do the same for the left and the right sides)

15 minutes of metabolic conditioning

Tuesday

Push-ups: 5 x 5

Pull-ups: 5 x 5

(Perform them as a *superset,* meaning you perform a set of five push-ups and then immediately perform a set of five pull-ups with no break. Repeat this for five sets.)

Goblet squats: 1, 2, 3, 4, 5, 1, 2, 3, 4, 5

Wednesday

Off

Thursday

Kettlebell swing practice set: 20 minutes (use a minimum of five reps per set)

Turkish get-up ladder: 1, 2, 3, 1, 2, 3

Pull-ups: 1, 2, 3, 1, 2, 3

15 minutes of metabolic conditioning

Friday

Dead lift: 1, 2, 3, 1, 2, 3

Goblet squats: 5 x 5

Push-ups: 1, 2, 3, 4, 5, 1, 2, 3, 4, 5

Saturday:

Off

Sunday

Off or 15 to 20 minutes of metabolic conditioning (optional)

Transforming Your Body with Metabolic Conditioning

The most powerful fat-burning weapon in your arsenal is metabolic conditioning. It has been proven, time and time again, that short and intense bouts of exercise are far more effective for burning fat, building muscle, and boosting natural growth hormone than long, trudging bouts of moderate-intensity exercise has ever been. And that's precisely what metabolic conditioning is about — short and sometimes varied bouts of intense exercise.

In these sections, we define metabolic conditioning, highlight some of its major benefits, and then help you choose the best method for metabolic conditioning to implement into your strength-training program.

Defining metabolic conditioning

Metabolic conditioning is simply an elevated cardiovascular stress plus moderate to heavy strength efforts. That is, metabolic conditioning, or *metcon,* blends strength and cardiovascular efforts in a short, intense, and compact bout of exercise.

To get a bit more into the science of it, the term *metabolic conditioning* actually refers to the training of the various metabolic systems in the human body that store and deliver energy, of which the three are as follows:

- ✔ **The phosphagen energy system (high power/short duration):** The *phosphagen energy system* fuels the most explosive and short-lived bouts of exercise, such as the first couple seconds of a sprint, a standing broad jump, or the swinging of a baseball bat.

- ✔ **The glycolytic energy system (moderate power/moderate duration):** The *glycolytic system* kicks in after the phosphagen system is spent and fuels moderately intense bouts of movement, such as most strength-training and weightlifting efforts.

- ✔ **The oxidative energy system (low power/long duration):** The *oxidative energy system* is the aerobic energy system; *aerobic* means with oxygen; the other two systems are *anaerobic,* meaning without oxygen. The oxidative energy system fuels lower-intensity and prolonged bouts of exercise, such as walking and distance running.

All three systems supply your body's molecular energy currency, *adenosine triphosphate,* or *ATP;* they just supply it at different rates. The phosphagen system, for example, supplies ATP quickly, but can only do so for a brief amount of time, whereas the oxidative system takes a little longer, but can supply ATP almost indefinitely. All your physical functions ultimately run on ATP.

The chief aim of metabolic conditioning is to increase the efficiency at which these systems store and deliver energy in the form of ATP — in simple words, to increase sheer work capacity — or the ability to do more physical work (both strength and cardiovascular) in the same amount or for longer periods of time.

Knowing when and how to do it

The good news: You can do metabolic conditioning training in many ways. Here are some of the most popular ways you can incorporate metabolic conditioning into your training plan:

Circuit training

Circuit training involves moving from various exercises and oftentimes equipment (body weight, barbells, kettlebells, and so on) with little to no rest in between. For example, a simple method is to move from five push-ups to five dead lifts to five pull-ups to five goblet squats without any rest between the exercises. ***Note:*** This method isn't an appropriate way to strength train, because fatigue will greatly limit the amount of weight you're able to lift. Fatigue is your friend for metabolic conditioning, but not for strength.

Circuit training is inherently fatiguing, which is pretty much the point. If you want to give circuit training a shot, start out by selecting three to five simple exercises (such as the kettlebell swing or the goblet squat) and perform them either for time (15 to 30 seconds each) or for reps (5 to 12 is a good range for metabolic circuit training). But whatever you choose, you must stop immediately if your form starts to sour. Any sort of *Olympic lifting* (such as the clean, jerk, and snatch), which we don't cover in this book, wouldn't be a good movement to include in circuit training, because these lifts are highly technical, demand a high level of concentration, and quickly fall apart under fatigue.

Interval training

Interval training involves exercising at various levels of intensity. Our favorite method of this is interval running, where you alternate between sprinting, jogging, and walking for a specified amount of time. For example, you can follow the sequence of 10 seconds of sprinting, 20 seconds of jogging, and 30 seconds of walking, repeated for 15 to 20 minutes.

Complex training

Complex training, or more specifically kettlebell complex training (which is our preferred method of metabolic conditioning), is similar to circuit training in the sense that it strings various exercises together (two or more), but does so using only a single instrument, such as kettlebells or barbells. What's unique about the kettlebell is that its compact design allows you to flow smoothly between movements without having to change weights or devices, which means you can get more work done in less time.

A kettlebell complex can be something as simple as combining kettlebell swings and goblet squats into a ladder format. For example:

> 2 kettlebell swings
>
> 1 goblet squat
>
> 4 kettlebell swings
>
> 2 goblet squats
>
> 6 kettlebell swings
>
> 3 goblet squats
>
> 8 kettlebell swings
>
> 4 goblet squat
>
> 10 kettlebell swings
>
> 5 goblet squats

Run that entire ladder without setting the kettlebell down and you'll quickly understand why kettlebell complex training is so effective for training metabolic conditioning and developing work capacity.

For the purposes of the program in the earlier section, "Looking at a sample week's workout," you should train metabolic conditioning twice per week, with an optional third session. Remember, do your metabolic training after your strength training, never before it (because you don't want fatigue to interfere with the quality of your strength training).

When deciding what specific type of metabolic training to do, you will benefit immensely by just starting with interval running. But if you want a little bit more variety, and perhaps some bigger bang for your buck, then check out all the kettlebell complexes that we provide in *Paleo Workouts For Dummies* (John Wiley & Sons, Inc.).

Killing Body Fat with Fasted Cardio: Take a Brisk Walk

One of the sneakiest ways to kill body fat dead is through *fasted cardio,* which means low-intensity aerobic activity, such as walking and hiking. While fasting, your body increases *lipolysis* (the releasing of fatty acids into the bloodstream). Fasted cardio can accelerate the *oxidation* (or burning off) of those fatty acids. The best time to take advantage is either first thing in the morning or immediately after your intense fasted workout session.

Get into the habit of fasted cardio first thing in the morning. Brew yourself a cup of green tea (it can help give you a little pep in the step, as well as intensify the fat-burning effects of fasting and low-intensity cardio), and then go for a brisk walk, a hike, or some other form of low-intensity cardio.

But fat burning is far from the only benefit of low-intensity cardiovascular activity. In these sections, we make the case for low-intensity cardio (LIC) and provide you with a few options on how to go about it.

Eyeing the many benefits of low-intensity cardio

In Taoist folklore, a monk supposedly lived beyond the age of 220 years. Although the truth of this account may be a bit stretched, this man undoubtedly existed, and undoubtedly lived well beyond 100 years old. And when asked what was his secret to his longevity, he simply replied, "brisk walking."

Low-intensity cardio has been shown to provide the following health benefits:

- Improved cardiovascular health
- Improved mood
- Stronger bones
- Weight (fat) loss
- Lower blood pressure
- Prevent diabetes
- Improved libido
- Stress reduction
- Reduced inflammation

We could go on and on with this list. Daily brisk walking for 20 to 30 minutes, more specifically daily brisk walking outdoors, and even more specifically daily brisk walking outdoors while fasting may very well be the single best thing you can do for your health.

Ditching the treadmill and doing what you love

You don't need a treadmill, the source of dread for many people, to do your low-intensity cardiovascular activity. If you enjoy walking, walk outside, preferably in minimalistic footwear (the less shoe, the better) because we want you to strengthen the small muscles in your feet and ankles. Most running shoes don't allow you to do so, because rather than strengthening, they compensate for weak feet or ankles.

What you do for your low-intensity cardio is limited only to your imagination and inspiration. Do what you love. If you love golf, then golf. If you love Frisbee, then play Frisbee. Just don't make the activity too intense. Keep what you do light and fun. You should be able to talk through it. If you find yourself gasping for air, you're probably pushing it a little too hard.

Even if you love the treadmill, we suggest you head outside and walk because the treadmill (especially when paired with overly cushy running shoes) promotes poor walking and running mechanics, which can lead to shin splints, knee problems, hip problems, and back problems. The list of injuries to be had from overworking by poor movement is limited only to the whole of the human anatomy. Just know that everything in the human body is connected, and if one thing goes out of order, all things can go out of order.

Chapter 13

Living the Fasting Lifestyle on a Daily Basis

● ●

In This Chapter

▶ Taking a look at the lifestyle patterns that will improve your fasting experience

▶ Getting the sleep and water you need to live lean, long, and strong

▶ Understanding the effects of stress on your body

▶ Eliminating toxins in your life to look and feel your best

● ●

*L*iving in this modern world brings many challenges. The way many people eat, move, and live has created a pandemic of chronic illnesses, so much so that these illnesses (such as diabetes, heart disease, and cancer) are now killing 80 percent of the industrialized world and are the leading causes of death. By 2017, chronic illness will cost $4.3 trillion per year in the United States alone!

What's so disheartening is that these chronic diseases are lifestyle-related diseases that can be prevented with the right choices. In fact, the greatest factor as to whether you'll be healthy and vibrant or sick and obese *is* your lifestyle choices. You're in the driver's seat. How your genes express themselves has much to do with the environment you choose to live in. In other words, your choices determine much of how good you look and feel.

Discovering the amazing ways you can get lean, healthy, and supercharged through fasting can absolutely make a big difference in your lifestyle. You'll go through life with fewer health challenges, and you'll look your best. But there's more to the picture. Lifestyle patterns are also an important part of your everyday living.

Lifestyle habits, such as managing stress, avoiding or reducing toxins, and realizing the value of water and sleep are all instrumental parts of your fasting regimen. This chapter walks you through some of those lifestyle patterns that are practical and important in helping you get the most out of your fasting and live a life that will keep you lean and strong, recharge you, and heal you.

Consuming More Water

Water is an essential part of fasting because of the *why* behind why fasting works; water gives the digestive system and many of the body functions a complete rest, and at the same time it enables the body to burn up and eliminate waste. To flush toxins out of your cells, your body needs water.

Drinking water is necessary because otherwise this burning up of debris in the system becomes too concentrated. In fact, without taking in water, you're apt to absorb some of the toxins or poisons that the debris may produce, which can defeat some of the benefits of drinking water that you can expect to achieve.

Drinking extra water also helps fat burning. Thinning the blood reduces the concentration of insulin in the blood, which gives a slight boost to the rate that fat cells expel fatty acids. (Refer to Chapter 2 for more on the science of insulin.)

The following sections take you through some of the important elements of water and explain why water is such a big deal. You also discover how to decode your body's signals in regards to hunger and thirst, and find out how to make sure your body is fueling up on water.

Grasping why water is so important

Fasting is a critical time to get water in your body, but even when you're not fasting, water is essential. In fact, your body consists of about 60 percent water. Just as your body needs *macronutrients* (such as healthy protein, carbohydrates, and fats) to function, it also needs water. Pure, clean water is the most essential of all nutrients. You can live for weeks without consuming food, but you can't go for more than a couple of days without water.

Proper intake of water is so vital to your well-being that deficiency of even 1 percent can present signs of dysfunctions in your body. Slightly more dehydration, and you have exponentially more health risks. You also need water to maintain the chemical balances in your body, such as these important functions:

- Balancing acid-base levels
- Eliminating waste from the lungs, skin, and colon (particularly during a fast)

    ✔ Regulating hormones

    ✔ Transporting nutrients to the cells

The minimum intake of water should be half of your body weight in ounces. However, when fasting, even more water is beneficial — just be mindful to keep drinking throughout the day and pay attention to thirst signals. So, for instance, if you weigh 150 pounds, then you should drink at least 75 ounces. If you're fasting, increase intake to around double that number, or 150 ounces. An easy way to gauge how well hydrated you are is to simply look at your urine. It should be fairly clear. If it's very dark yellow, that's a sign you may need to drink more water.

Your body responds with different signals when it's dehydrated or hungry. Many times, people read the signs wrong and intervene with food, medicines, or procedures that aren't necessary. Sometimes, all your body really needs is some water — another one of those simple health weapons that's often overlooked because it seems so simple.

Recognizing your thirst button

Listening to your body when it comes to thirst is really important, especially when you're fasting. Getting enough water helps minimize the sensation of hunger and keeps the toxins moving out of the body. Recognize that what you may think is hunger during a fast may very well be thirst.

Here's how it works: Your brain recognizes low energy levels available for body functions, including hunger and thirst. Because brain signals are simultaneous, people sometimes confuse these signals and assume they need food when they actually need water. One of the main problems with this confusion between thirst and hunger is not understanding how much water you really need and misinterpreting the signs of dehydration. The key is to be attuned with your body and know when to drink water. You can do this by simply doing the urine test. Your urine should be fairly clear. If it's very dark yellow, that's a sign you may need to drink more water.

The biggest roadblock is waiting until you're thirsty to drink. Your brain center doesn't send a message until you're almost 2 percent dehydrated. By then, you've likely already encountered some problems associated with dehydration. Your kidneys receive the low signal before you do, and they respond by decreasing urine output, a big sign that you need more water.

How do you know whether you're dehydrated? You guessed it: the urine test. If you're not urinating at least six to eight times a day and your urine is dark yellow, you need more water.

Here's how some of the signs of dehydration play out in your system:

- ✔ Excess body weight
- ✔ Chronic hunger
- ✔ High blood pressure
- ✔ High blood cholesterol
- ✔ Headaches
- ✔ Depression
- ✔ Intestinal pain
- ✔ Arthritis pain

TIP

One of the best ways to prevent dehydration is to pre-hydrate in the morning! It gets your blood moving and transports all the good stuff to where your body needs it!

REMEMBER

Dial into your body's signal. When you're not feeling well, having low energy, or feeling hungry, your first line of defense is always drink water. It's easy in this fast-paced world to let your tank get too low.

Keeping the water you drink clean

Because you're focusing on fasting, which removes toxins from your body, the last thing you want to do is add more toxins with the water you drink. Tap water is easy to get and low in cost. But is it healthy to drink? Unless you know your tap water is safe, drink it only when you're desperate, and look for a cleaner source.

The Environmental Working Group (EWG) obtained almost 20 million records from state water officials. Its conclusion was that the U.S. federal government should perform a national assessment of drinking water. Incredibly, more than half of the chemical pollutants the group found (315 total) aren't subject to any health or safety regulations, so they can show up in your water in any amount, and it's legal.

The contaminants you have to be concerned about in tap water are as follows:

- ✔ Bacteria
- ✔ Environmental chemicals
- ✔ Heavy metals

- ✔ Parasites
- ✔ Radiological pollution

Also, public water systems, where the water is filtered, add chlorine and fluoride back into the water. You also have to think about your home's pipes. The type of pipes you have and any corrosion can cause contamination.

To make a decision about whether your water is safe, you may have to do some investigation. If you have a public water system, you have the right to ask for the results from past water tests. The Environmental Protection Agency (EPA) requires utilities to provide a consumer confidence report. If you have well water, you'll have to have it tested yourself.

Having your water tested by a laboratory takes away all the guesswork. Your local health authority may offer free test kits. For a great resource on certified testing labs and water in your area, call the EPA's drinking water hot line (800-426-4791) or go to www.water.epa.gov/hotline/index.cfm. The EWG also has an information site where you can see how your state's water ranks at www.ewg.org/tap-water/home.

Choosing clean water

One of the simplest ways you can make a difference in your fasting outcome to lose weight and get healthier is to listen to your body — and choose to drink clean, pure water. You may not have access to pure stream or river water, but you can get close.

Your body needs pure, clean water without chorine, fluoride, and toxins. The best way to get this kind of water is through a water filtration system. Knowing what's in your water and what needs to be filtered out is a good place to start, and this is where water testing comes in (see the preceding section).

If you don't want to test your water, at the very least, make sure the filtration removes the following:

- ✔ Arsenic
- ✔ Chlorine
- ✔ Chloroform
- ✔ *E. coli*
- ✔ Fluoride
- ✔ Nitrites and nitrates
- ✔ Radon

You can choose from a system that filters the water in one area of your house or a whole-house filtration system. The best-case scenario is to make sure all the water in your house is filtered, including bath water and cooking water. Choose a system that fits your personal needs and budget.

Don't replace drinking water from the tap with bottled water. Water bottles aren't an alternative because the plastic packaging pollutes your body and the world. The chemical Bisphenol A (BPA) and phthalates contained in plastics are dangerous to your health. Even low levels of these chemicals cause disease and can create hormonal disturbances. Also, 40 percent of bottled water is simply taken from municipal tap water, so most bottled water is really nothing more than tap water in toxic bottles.

Simplifying Stress

Your body goes through somewhat of a stressful process when you're fasting through reduced energy availability. Your body adapts to this mild stress of not having food by functioning at a higher level by better regulating glucose, becoming more sensitive to insulin, and burning fat. In order for this process to work its best, though, reducing any other stressors in your life (such as work-related stress) is essential.

The less stress you put yourself through, the more energy your body will have to deal with the positive short-term stress that will help you burn fat, heal, and regenerate. These sections help you discover your body's responses to stress, so you can take steps to manage your stress.

Examining your body's response to stress

Your body isn't designed to be under chronic stress. In fact, your body has a built-in system called the *sympathetic nervous system,* also referred to as the *fight or flight response,* which activates in times of stress. This mechanism helps your body when you're in moments of crisis (for example, a tiger chasing you).

With modern-day living, people constantly stimulate this system, which is most definitely not how this system was designed to be used. This constant triggering causes problems that can lead to even bigger problems.

When you're under chronic stress, you force your body to adapt to whatever the crisis situation is. The physiological stress expresses itself in many ways. When you're fasting, your body has even more difficulty dealing with stressors, because you ideally want your body to be working at cleansing your cells and burning fat and not dealing with other challenges.

Here are some of the symptoms of chronic stress adaptation:

- ✔ Anxiety
- ✔ Blood sugar problems
- ✔ Decreased fertility
- ✔ Decreased growth hormone
- ✔ Depression
- ✔ Fatigue
- ✔ High blood pressure
- ✔ Hormonal changes
- ✔ Increased heart rate
- ✔ Memory problems
- ✔ Obesity

 The best way to get well, stay well, and have the life you want is to remove chronic stressors from your life. Remove yourself from whatever physiological or environmental factors are causing these stressors and put yourself in an environment (whatever that means to you) that is free of constant stress. We know that removing yourself from the stress is sometimes easier said than done. If you need help, ask family members, friends, coworkers, or professionals. Eliminating the stress will be helpful to any fast, as well as make a big improvement in the quality of your life everyday.

 When you get stressed, you may sometimes turn to medications; however, they're not the solution. Your very intelligent innate system, which you were born with, is doing exactly what it's supposed to do in response to stress. The symptoms or diseases you have occur because your body is expressing your chronic stress.

Seeing the link between stress and belly fat

One of the amazing things about fasting is its ability to burn fat. For people who have had terrible weight-loss resistance, finally seeing the needle move on the scale is really liberating. Stress, however, interferes with some of the most stubborn fat — belly fat.

Belly fat is resistant fat, sometimes coined *the middle-aged spread*. It's the dangerous midsection fat that flops over your jeans. If you want to do away with stubborn belly fat, you have to address the stressors in your life. Maintaining the right attitude, the food you choose, and the relationships you chose to be in are important. You also need to eliminate environmental factors, such as toxins (refer to the later section, "Taking on Toxins" for more information) and exercise more to reduce stress levels.

Belly fat isn't the cause of all diseases. Your body adapts to the stressors that cause the belly fat. So, in the end, your stressors are actually causing the diseases. Your belly fat is only a symptom.

As your stress rises, so do your stress hormones, such as *cortisol.* When your stress hormones rise and your feel-good hormone *(serotonin)* decreases, it's disastrous. The result of this combination includes the following symptoms:

- Depression
- Drop in growth hormone
- Exhaustion
- Insomnia
- Insulin problems
- Weight gain

One of the best actions you can take to get rid of dangerous, unattractive belly fat is to reduce your stress. Create an environment that allows your body to express its fullest potential. Find ways to reduce your stress and you'll have more success with your fasting. Chapter 3 offers some suggestions to help you reach the right mindset and focus your attention on yourself and your fasting lifestyle.

Getting Enough Sleep: Your Body's Weapon

Sleep is always critically important — whether fasting or not, but even more so when you're fasting because your body needs to regenerate more then ever, and this regeneration happens while you sleep. Sleep also suppresses your appetite (making fasting easier).

Many people report that they're shocked at how much better they're sleeping when fasting. It's one of the best side effects of fasting and what happens when the structures and functions of your body begin to heal and regenerate.

If sleep has been a challenge for you, then fasting can make a big difference. These sections help you discover the shocking truth of what happens when you're short on sleep and give some tips on getting the best shut-eye you possibly can. Nothing makes you feel more powerful than sound sleep, and between fasting and these tips, it will definitely make a difference in helping you perform better during the day.

Falling short of sleep

So many things interfere with sleep today: Emails, TVs with 150 channels, more hobbies, social media, and smartphones have all become such a part of living in today's modern world that people borrow time from sleep to do more. A lack of sleep can accumulate and before long, sleep deprivation sets in, which leads to a host of serious problems.

Sleep deprivation isn't a joke. When you lack sleep, here are some potential outcomes that may startle you:

- **Illness:** Not getting enough sleep doubles your rate of breast cancer and other diseases. The best sleep pattern for a person to follow is to go to bed by 10 p.m. and wake no later then 7 a.m. The sleep you get before midnight does a lot to regenerate your body, and waking early is your body's sleep-awake cycle.

- **Weight gain:** Sleep deprivation causes you to gain weight. Proper sleep helps you lose weight. In fact, you can lose 14.3 pounds a year by getting one more hour of sleep a night.

- **Hormonal shifts:** When you don't get enough sleep, hormones shift, causing your appetite to change. The sugars you crave increase your insulin, creating blood sugar problems. These hormonal shifts cause weight gain and health issues.

- **Heart disease:** When your hormones shift, causing you to eat more sugar, you get insulin resistance (see Chapter 2). Insulin resistance can cause weight gain. During this process, you convert all your carbohydrates into bad cholesterol and you retain water, which alters your blood pressure and paves the way to heart disease.

- **Lowered immune system:** The body's immune system is weakened without sleep. The number of white cells in your body actually decreases.

- **Altered brainpower:** Memory, concentration, and creativity are all impaired with lack of sleep.

- **Premature aging:** The body decreases its growth hormone needed for ongoing tissue repair, healing, cell rejuvenation, and bone function. Growth hormone can reverse the affects of aging; therefore, sleep deprivation causes aging.

- ✔ **Sugar handling problems:** When you're sleep-deprived, the ability to metabolize sugar decreases, turning sugar into fat.

- ✔ **Decreased regenerative powers:** Sleep is needed to regenerate the body, especially the brain. When you don't have enough sleep, your body doesn't heal or regenerate.

- ✔ **Prolonged high cortisol levels:** When you're awake for long periods of time with the lights on, the hormone cortisol doesn't naturally drop like it's supposed to. High cortisol occurs in nature when you need it to run fast or deal with pain from an injury. This constant high cortisol causes people to become panicky and depressive.

- ✔ **Cumulative effect:** Sleep deprivation is cumulative. You don't adapt to sleep deprivation; you only get more tired and, eventually, unhealthy and overweight.

Creating a natural rhythm

Getting in the habit of training your body to sleep during its natural rhythm is key. You want to sleep during the darkness and awake when it's light. Staying up all night in artificial light confuses your system.

When you constantly trick your *circadian rhythm* (your body's natural sleep cycle during a 24-hour period) by staying up too long in artificial light, your body thinks it's a long summer day. What your body naturally expects to follow is the cold, short days of winter. The concern, however, is that the expected dormant hibernation period after the long summer never comes, which makes your mind start to literally go crazy. Nature thinks you're up too long, that you've eaten more than your share of nature's goodness, and that you're likely infertile from being bathed in insulin. Your body creates a bipolar state of mind, and you become depressive and manic.

Also, when the light never dims, your cortisol never drops. Chronic high cortisol and chronic high insulin put your mind in a chronic state of panic. When insulin and cortisol are too high or too low, more than just moodiness occurs; you experience true manic depression and mental illness.

The National Institute of Mental Health agrees that one of the primary causes of depression and mental illness is simply being out of sync with the dark-light rhythm that your body expects. Most of the drugs for depression are aimed at putting your sleep cycles back in place.

Start looking at sleep as a nutrient. As much as you look at evolutionary eating, moving, and living as your blueprint, staying in tune with your natural sleep design is just as essential.

Sleep works together with all other areas in your life to provide you the best health. Here are a few tips for getting the right amount and quality of sleep you need:

- **Go to bed at the same time every night.** If you don't give yourself a scheduled bedtime, you get distracted. Before long, your awake time will be squeezing its way into your much-needed sleep time.

- **Go to bed by no later than 10 p.m. and wake up by no later than 7 a.m.** Set your phone, watch, or an alarm clock to remind you to close down shop for the night. Most of your body's repairing goes on before 1 a.m., and you get more growth hormone. Your circadian rhythm will also be in sync with your sleep-awake cycle.

- **Rise with the sun.** The sunlight will regulate your hormones for the day.

- **Unplug.** Make sure you're not doing anything but relaxing, journaling, or reading one to two hours before bed. This quiet time releases the hormone *melatonin* to get you to sleep. That means no TV, no computer, or anything stimulating. Dim the lights if you can. Doing so allows your body to start producing even more melatonin. Move all alarm clocks or electrical devices at least 3 feet away from your bed.

- **Black out your bedroom room completely.** Your body produces melatonin in darkness. Cover the windows to prevent any light from coming in. Use blackout shades if you need to. You shouldn't be able to see even your hand in front of your face. If your room is too light when you try to sleep, hormone production slows down.

- **Keep your room cool and well ventilated.** Keep your room at a temperature that's comfortable for you, but make sure it's on the cooler side — about 68 degrees works for most people. Some people also like an air purifier. Using one can improve the way you breathe and, ultimately, the way you sleep.

- **Limit caffeine.** Drinking caffeine prolongs the time it takes you to go to sleep and decreases the amount of deep sleep you get. The time it takes for about half of the caffeine you've had to clear out of your system is three to five hours, so plan accordingly. Caffeine limitations vary greatly from person to person, so see what works for you.

- **Limit alcohol:** Alcohol may make you fall asleep quicker, but your quality of sleep is diminished. Deep sleep and REM sleep, which stands for Rapid Eye Movement, are both greatly reduced, so even if you fall asleep more quickly, you'll probably wake up feeling tired. (During REM sleep, most of your muscles become paralyzed, and your brain's activity becomes quite intense, similar to the activity during wakefulness. Most people are able to have vivid dreams during REM sleep.)

Make sleep as essential as fasting, eating healthy foods, exercising, or anything else you do that you consider important to your health (and waistline).

Sleep-inducing foods include turkey and almonds as well as seasonings like nutmeg, turmeric, and garlic. (Try herbal tea with nutmeg, or turkey broth with garlic as a before-bed snack to prep for a restful night.)

Taking on Toxins

Ridding your body of toxins is one of the cornerstones of fasting. Eliminating toxins can help you think more clearly, burn fat, boost immunity, make you look younger, and perform better at everything you do.

Pay attention to all kinds of toxins around you and try to reduce them as much as possible. You can tap into the benefits of being toxin-free the more you identify where toxins are lingering and how you can reduce them from your life.

When your surroundings are toxin-free, so are you. Here are some of the benefits:

- More energy
- Bright, sparkly eyes
- Clear skin
- Weight loss
- Less pain
- Deepened sense of spirituality

These sections explain how you can eliminate toxins in your home and in your body.

Society's chemical culture

Many people are walking around sick and frustrated because they can't get answers to why they're chronically fatigued and unwell. With blood tests and exams revealing normal results, it can make someone feel lost. For years, this chronic, unexplained fatigue was thought to be just "all in their head," but now, scientists and doctors understand that many illnesses and unexplained fatigue may be the results of toxins in the system (called the *toxic burden*).

The amount of toxins around you is jaw-dropping. For instance, studies by the National Resource Defense Council state that the use of pesticides is ten times what it was in the 1940s. In the United States alone, more than 1.2 billion pounds of pesticides are used per year. At least 70,000 chemicals are used in businesses today, 6 trillion pounds annually.

Identifying toxins in the home

Enhance your fast by removing as many toxins from the home as you can. Toxins in your home include any pollutants that are in your daily surroundings.

Here are some common toxins and what to do about them:

- **Cleaning solutions:** Cleaning products can be hazardous because you inhale chemicals in the fumes that these products often give off. Drain openers, air fresheners, ammonia-based cleaners, and chlorine bleach all contain toxins. These toxins are neurotoxic chemicals, meaning that they're damaging to your nervous system. The good news is that many nontoxic cleaners are widely available, so you don't need to use neurotoxic chemicals to clean your house. Try an all-natural cleaner or use some old-fashioned ingredients, like borax, baking soda, vinegar, soap, and water.

- **Indoor air:** Most people spend 90 percent of their time indoors, so air quality is paramount. However, the Environmental Protection Agency (EPA) says that indoor air is two to five times more polluted than outside air because of the chemical products people use, which they come in contact with and inhale.

  To reduce toxins from indoor air, you can do a couple things:

  - **Get some good ol' fresh air:** Make sure you allow your home to get fresh air every day. Crack open the windows just enough to permit airflow. When it's really cold, just open them for five minutes, and it'll still help.

  - **Buy a good air purifier:** You want the purifier to filter bacteria, molds, toxic fumes, smoke, dust, dander, pollens, static electricity, and hydrocarbons (from cooking). You can find great units at most home improvement stores.

- **Dry cleaning:** Keeping your dry cleaning to a minimum can keep your home and your skin healthier. See the next section, "Eliminating toxins from your body" for more information.

- **Carpets, rugs, and furniture:** Carpeting is heavily sprayed with insecticides. Toxic carpets are one of the most dangerous toxins you can have because you're exposed to them all day and all night. You can reduce toxins in carpets or rugs by airing them outside for a few days before you place them in your home. Also, instead of wall-to-wall carpets, opt for area rugs to reduce toxins. Always look for natural fibers, such as wool-cotton blend, and make sure they don't have a latex backing.

Look for the Carpet and Rug Institute (CRI) low-emission labels before buying (www.carpet-rug.org/commercial-customers/cleaning-and-maintenance/seal-of-approval-products).

Eliminating toxins from your body

Your skin is your largest organ. Yes, your skin is actually an organ, and anything you put on the skin has a direct route into your bloodstream. When you put something on your skin, ask yourself, "Is this product pure enough that I could actually eat it?" If not, you probably shouldn't have it on your skin at all.

You can make toxin-free choices with these common products:

- **Makeup and moisturizers:** Makeup and moisturizers include numerous chemicals. A good way to find toxin-free options is to purchase unscented brands. They usually have no petrochemicals or their derivatives. Look for a company that makes it a priority not to use harmful ingredients.

- **Perfumes:** Perfumes can cause toxins and allergies in many people. Instead, try essential oils, which are lightly fragranced in different scents. You can even buy them in sprays or roll-ons. Most health food stores and grocers carry essential oils.

- **Antiperspirants:** Stay away from any antiperspirants that have aluminum in them. Because you're putting these products under your arm near the breast tissue, you need to be extra cautious. You shouldn't put anything with toxins near your breast tissue. Opt for a more natural deodorant, which doesn't contain aluminum. This holds true for both men and women.

- **Nail polish:** Nail products are filled with chemicals. Actually, a nail spa can be a toxic trap if your provider uses products with chemicals. Look for holistic spas where you have a better chance of getting a more natural product (and a better experience all around).

- **Toothpastes:** Toothpastes are often filled with toxins, and some even contain artificial sugars. Opt for a more natural brand, like Tom's of Maine, where you don't have to worry about all the chemicals and toxins included on the label.

- **Shampoos:** Take a minute and read the back of your shampoo bottle. We bet you can't even say half of the ingredients. Shampoos have tons of chemicals. You can find alternatives pretty easily if you look. For example, Aveda is a good option and widely available.

Your body is a beautiful intelligent system. It renews and regenerates when you give it the raw material to do so. You're part of the world, and the world is part of you. You have to work within this framework to reduce toxins the best you can.

Although this information may be daunting, the marketplace is seeing more and more toxin-free foods and products every year. As awareness increases, so will the choices. Make sure you educate yourself on where you can cut back on your daily surroundings of toxins and select different choices that fit your needs. When you shift your paradigm to wellness, you get better as you go along, and making better choices becomes fluid after you've done it for a while.

Part V
The Part of Tens

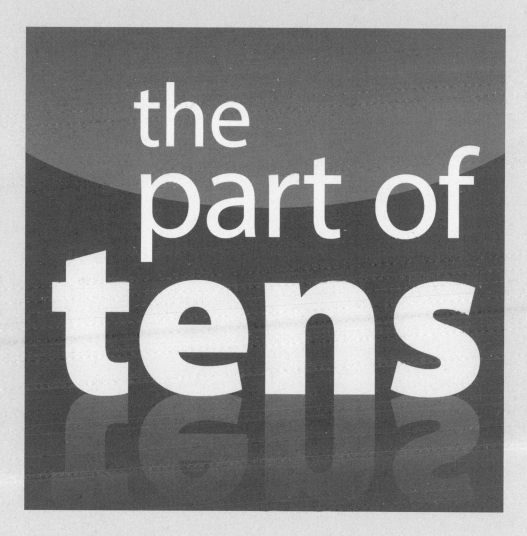

Visit www.dummies.com/extras/fastdiets for a bonus Part of Tens list for more tips to help you succeed with your fast.

In this part...

- ✔ Grasp the concept of hunger and how accepting it will ultimately help you succeed at fasting — and help you enjoy eating that much more.

- ✔ Discover how recreation, play, and exercise can optimize your fasts — from keeping your energy high to burning fat and building muscle.

- ✔ See how visualization can help you achieve successful fasts and a new healthier lifestyle.

- ✔ Comprehend the ways in which common beverages, such as green tea and coffee — not expensive supplements — can enhance a fast through antioxidant absorption, increased fat loss, and appetite control.

- ✔ Understand how meditation can serve multiple purposes in your fasting lifestyle — from staving off hunger to keeping you motivated.

Chapter 14

Ten Ways to Stave Off Hunger

In This Chapter

▶ Understanding how to keep hunger at bay while fasting

▶ Discovering fun and productive ways to keep your mind off food

▶ Drinking water, tea, and coffee to suppress hunger and amplify your fast

*H*unger doesn't make fasting difficult. Your reaction to the hunger does. If at the first sign of hunger you seek out food, you need to ask yourself an important question: Do you control your hunger, or does your hunger control you?

Fasting is a discipline, and discipline is much like a muscle. It grows stronger the more you use it. But with fasting, you don't work against weight. Instead, to grow your fasting muscle, you have to work against hunger. By controlling your hunger, you can strengthen your fasting practice.

Recognize the hunger from fasting for what it truly is — the dying of bad habits and the disappearing of desires. Your hunger while fasting isn't a physiological need for nutrition but simply a craving. True hunger brought about by long-term deprivation, deficiencies, or starvation isn't the same as the hunger you feel from skipping a few meals — not even close.

However, we do admit that just sitting around and doing nothing with your hunger is a tough task, and one that sets you up for fasting failure. So in this chapter, we give you ten strategies to stave off hunger and keep productive throughout your fasting period.

Accept It

The most important aspect of controlling hunger is to accept it. Acknowledge before you begin your fast that hunger will rear its ugly head, and that it won't hurt you; it will only try to intimidate you.

Being hungry from time to time is good and natural because it's a way of knowing that you're doing the right thing. Hunger is a primal instinct — it provides impetus and motivation, which you can only achieve in a fasted state. Many anthropologists believe that humans should naturally be hungry during the day, and in a fed and relaxed state in the evening, because it matches up with humanity's natural biorhythms and flow between sympathetic (fight or flight) and parasympathetic (rest and digest) nervous systems. If you're never hungry, then you have a problem.

Fasting and feeding is yin and yang. The human body needs a balance between the two for optimal health. Most people clearly suffer from too much yang (feeding) and not enough yin (fasting).

Drink Plenty of Water

The simplest, easiest, and healthiest method to stave off hunger while fasting is to consume adequate amounts of fluid, especially water. Much of the time, hunger is actually thirst — so you should reach for some water. In fact, filling up on good, clean water will be your number one weapon to combat hunger.

Although the recommended amount of water is eight glasses (or 64 ounces) per day, Americans fall far short of this amount, drinking only two-and-a-half glasses (or 20 ounces) per day, which is 58 gallons of water, on average, a year. In comparison, the average American also consumes 44 gallons of soda annually. In your quest to become truly healthful, cutting the amount of soda down to zero gallons would be wise.

The truth is you can actually derive close to a sufficient amount of water through a proper diet. However, when you're fasting, you must increase your water intake to compensate. The general rule is to drink more water than you're used to. We suggest carrying around a container of water at all times, to regularly sip from. And whenever your hunger swells to the point of severe distraction and hindrance, go have a tall glass of water.

Drinking any water isn't enough. You also want to be selective with your water. Not all water is created equal, so go the extra mile and spend the extra penny to ensure that your water is clean and free of harmful contaminants as far as practicable. Buy a water filtration system for your home, if possible, or opt for bottled water such as Kiwaii, which is true spring water and comes in BPA-free plastic. Stay away from most public drinking water because it's a cesspool of toxic waste, brimming with harmful chemicals, toxins, and hormones.

Grab a Cup of Tea or Coffee

Caffeine and other nervous system stimulants often function to suppress hunger. Having a cup of organic tea or coffee to start your day or right after a workout can keep hunger from knocking on your door. That cup can wage a pre-emptive strike against hunger, hydrating the system, boosting energy levels, and at the same time delivering a delectable surge of antioxidants.

Caffeinated teas, such as green tea, black tea, or pu-erh tea, and coffee promote a feeling of being full and satisfied, not only though increased fluid intake, but also with a moderate influx of caffeine. Caffeine, in moderation, comes with a number of notable benefits, including:

- ✔ Improved cognitive function (memory)
- ✔ Decreased hunger
- ✔ Increased fat burning
- ✔ Increased energy levels
- ✔ Decreased risk of Alzheimer's disease
- ✔ Decreased muscle soreness after exercise
- ✔ Increased stamina during exercise

Coffee can actually ward off hunger more aggressively than tea because the caffeine content in most coffees is higher than the content in most teas.

Caffeine is a powerful substance and harmful in unregulated doses. Too much caffeine reverses many of the positive benefits to be had from moderate caffeine consumption and brings along a number of negative side effects including heart palpitations, restlessness, anxiety, and even insomnia. Do your best to keep caffeine intake at or under two cups of tea or coffee per day (that's less than two ventis at Starbucks).

If you determine that two cups aren't doing it for you anymore, meaning you're not getting the same positive and stimulatory boost that you used to, then eliminate coffee altogether and allow your system to reset for a month. Then slowly add back your cup or two of coffee. This natural cycling of coffee ensures that you remain sensitive to its effects and get the most from the minimum dose.

Don't consume coffee or any other sort of stimulatory agent after noon, unless you plan on staying up way past your bedtime. And if you do notice that you're having trouble sleeping, either push your coffee consumption to early in the day, consume less of it, or both.

Do Some Household Chores or Gardening

Another good way to keep your mind off hunger is to engage in some household chores or do some gardening. They both are productive distractions, and your family will appreciate all the wonderful work you've done!

Household chores, such as cleaning, or gardening keep you focused on something other than your hunger as well as help you maintain a cleaner more organized home and manicured yard. And there's nothing quite like growing your own food, because it's healthy, rewarding, and delicious.

If you don't like to garden, no big deal. You can tackle other chores around the house, as we're sure your partner has told you many times. Now you have no excuse. There's no better time to get around to doing them while in a fasted state.

Work

To keep your mind off your hunger, you can also perform some work-related tasks that you've been putting off, such as finishing that report, responding to some emails, and so on. For your fast to be productive, you have to keep your mind focused anywhere else but on your hunger. The busier you are, the easier your fast will be, in most cases.

No matter what type of job you have, focus on how you can do your job better (and then do it) while you're fasting. Set yourself to a task that will keep you busy and distracted. Sitting around with your hunger and doing nothing is only going to make the whole fasting process far more difficult than it ought to be.

Go for a Walk

Walking briskly maximizes the fat-burning effects to be had when you're fasting. A brisk walk also promotes a healthy heart and supports your overall well-being. Brisk walking is without a doubt one of the healthiest things you can do. And, so is fasting. So go ahead and combine the two.

Brisk walking, like most other forms of exercise, can also help to keep your hunger levels low. It does so not only by providing an enjoyable distraction, but also by encouraging your body to start burning stored body fat as a means for energy.

Play Some Sports or Enjoy a Hobby

Any and all physical activity is going to enhance the positive effects of fasting, as long as you don't overdo it. If you have a favorite recreational sport, such as tennis, pickup basketball, or ultimate Frisbee, or any other sort of physical hobby, then we encourage you to engage in it throughout your fasting period.

Playing a sport and engaging in physical activity is a good way to trick your body into fasting and exercise because your mind is focused not on the exercising or the fasting, but on the activity itself. The physical activity is merely a side effect of play.

Even nonphysical hobbies, such as knitting, playing a musical instrument, painting, reading, or basket weaving, can be a great diversion. And although we love movement, and advocate it as much as possible, there is nothing wrong with keeping yourself distracted with hobbies that don't require much in the way of physical exertion. Although not physically vexing, they're mentally stimulating and beneficial in their own right.

Engage in Some Short, Intense Exercise

Engaging in bouts of short and intense exercise throughout your fasting period is an obvious way to keep your mind from thinking about your hunger. Intense exercise, such as weight lifting or sprinting, suppresses hunger, boosts muscle, and blasts fat.

Twenty to 30 minutes of intense exercise toward the end of your fasting period is ideal. Even more ideal is to tack on another 20 to 30 minutes of brisk walking after the intense exercise before you eat. Refer to Chapter 12 for specific exercises that you can try.

Meditate

Meditation allows you to sit still, relax, and control your thinking, and in turn, control your stress and anxiety. It's a powerful agent to aid in the battle against any demon (in this case, hunger) that you may be facing. Although meditation isn't the easiest method to suppress hunger, it does work, and over time, as you get better at meditation, you'll get better at accepting your hunger, perhaps even embracing it.

Meditation, like intense exercise, is often best performed in short, but frequent bouts. It takes a practiced and disciplined meditator to effectively meditate for longer periods of time. Ten to 15 minutes, two to four times a day is a good start. You can use meditation to sit with your hunger, accept it, and figure out how to underreact to it, rather than overreact to it.

To discover more about how to meditate, check out *Meditation For Dummies* by Stephan Bodian and Dean Ornish, MD (John Wiley & Sons, Inc.).

Munch on Some Live Foods

If you must eat throughout the fasting period and simply can't control your hunger, then your best option is to enter into a *controlled fast,* which is the premise behind the undereating phase of the Warrior Diet. (Refer to Chapter 7 for more details about the Warrior Diet.)

With a controlled fast, you eat lightly throughout the fast, and by lightly, we mean foods that tax the digestive system very little. As a result, you need to eat a small quantity and select the right foods. You should ideally eat only *live* fruits and vegetables, which are foods with the *lowest glycemic index* (those foods that have the smallest impact on your blood sugar levels) and foods that haven't been cooked. Cooking kills the natural enzymes contained within food that aids in its digestion. If you choose to practice a controlled fast, then you may have some light, live foods every couple of hours. Chapter 2 explains in greater depth how foods with a lower glycemic index can benefit your goals.

Here are some examples of live food you can eat during a controlled fast:

- ✔ Green and cruciferous vegetables, such as broccoli.

- ✔ Root vegetables, such as carrots and ginger. In fact, fresh carrot and ginger juice is one of the best natural detoxifiers to aid in a fast.

- ✔ Thin-skinned fruits, which are primarily berries, such as blueberries, blackberries, raspberries, and strawberries. Don't overconsume them. A handful is more than plenty.

Any full meal is automatically disqualified and immediately throws you out of a state of natural detoxification, which is what you're attempting to derive from a controlled fast.

Chapter 15

Ten Ways to Stay Motivated

*F*asting has many, many benefits. By following any of the fasting methods we outline in Part II, you can set yourself on the path to health. But sometimes even knowing all the benefits of a healthy lifestyle doesn't mean that you'll be able to stay motivated all the time to adhere to that lifestyle. So in this chapter, we discuss different techniques you can use to get and stay motivated.

You don't have to stick with just one of these motivational tactics. In fact, if you employ a combination of any of them, you can increase your chances of success. Figure out which ones work best for you and practice them.

Find a Fasting Accountabili-buddy

Research has shown that enlisting a friend, or an *accountabili-buddy* as we like to call it, to join you in a healthy lifestyle overhaul will set you up for greater success. You'll lose more weight, and you'll stick with the program longer than if you had gone it alone.

Choose an accountabili-buddy who can help you stay positive and on track, someone who can provide you with the support you need to get through any distractions or temptations, even the 15 minutes you spend pining for a cookie from the tray that your coworker brought into the office. And in turn, you'll feel satisfaction knowing that you can provide similar support at those times when you're motivated and the other person isn't as much.

Given today's widely connected world, the friend that you pick doesn't have to be local. Maybe a Facebook friend who lives across the country wants to join you in your lifestyle change or perhaps you want to join an online forum or community. Your accountabili-buddy doesn't have to be just one person either. You may rely on a number of people whom you have come to know via their own posts on those forums. In fact, becoming active in an online community can be a very effective method to getting the support you'll sometimes need in order to stay motivated.

No matter who your accountabili-buddy is or where he or she lives, having a friend (or virtual friends) on call who can help motivate you on those days when you just can't motivate yourself will go a long way in keeping you successful in your healthy lifestyle journey.

Read Articles/Blogs or Watch Videos

Sometimes all you need to get or stay motivated is to watch or read something that inspires you. Reading a blog or various articles or watching a video clip about someone else's successful body and lifestyle transformations can be very powerful and go a long way in making you feel up to the task of sticking with your new healthy lifestyle.

If you frequent a blog or website that you know helps you get or stay motivated, keep it bookmarked on your web browser, smartphone, or tablet for easy access whenever you need that little spark. If you don't know of one, you can download many applications on your smartphone or tablet to help you with motivation.

 A quick search can identify motivational apps that you can download (many for free) and keep on hand for those times when you're in need of a little inspiration. If you don't have a smartphone or tablet, you can also use an online search engine or go on www.youtube.com and look for "keep me motivated" materials.

Just be sure and find something that motivates you for the *right* reasons. You want to cultivate positive motivation, not feel bad about yourself, so choose wisely. Plenty of great resources to get inspired are out there; you just need to find the ones that work best for you.

Set a Short-Term Goal with a Reward

Choose a goal that you can measure and attain in a relatively short amount of time, and after you reach that goal, reward yourself with something that isn't related to junk food. And when we say a short amount of time, we really do mean short! Maybe your goal focuses on successfully making it through a day or two.

No matter how far — or near — into the future you set that goal, make sure you can clearly see the end. Make the goal very explicit. For instance, instead of saying, "I will get fit," set very definable parameters, such as "I will fast for 16 hours today." That way, you know exactly what success looks like, and even better, you know without a doubt that you earned your reward.

Although some people may use food as the ultimate reward for a job well done, we suggest you treat yourself to an experience, such as a massage, which is a healthier option. Other options include going shopping and purchasing new workout clothes or a new blender to juice fruits and veggies. You don't have to spend money though. You can go on a walk and reflect on how amazing you now feel after reaching your goal. Get creative, and discover what healthy rewards motivate you most when you need that motivation the most.

If you make food your ultimate reward, then you'll constantly feel like you're depriving yourself when you aren't eating those rewarding foods. Instead, choose a reward that is meaningful to you but that doesn't involve sabotaging the progress you've made.

Recognize That Sometimes You Need a Carrot and Sometimes You Need a Stick

Rewarding yourself may not do the trick to keep motivated quite as well as if you "punished" yourself for not completing a goal. With this motivational tactic, we certainly don't advocate beating yourself up. Instead, we suggest that the stick you use is accountability.

No matter what motivation tools you choose to use from this chapter, you want to set an attainable and measurable goal. After you have your specific goal and deadline, you next need to decide what you have to do if you don't meet your goal. Maybe you decide that you have to do a chore you normally can't stand, or you can't have whatever reward you would've received had you succeeded. (Refer to Chapter 3 for specific ways to set realistic expectations and goals.)

Don't use deprivation as an anti-reward (we mean for instance not to punish yourself with an extra fasting day that week). In the same manner, don't use exercise as the stick, either, such as making yourself do a hundred push-ups because you didn't meet your goal. Even though the goals may be nutrition or fitness-based, don't make the anti-rewards nutrition or fitness-based. Leading a healthy lifestyle means that eating well, fasting, exercising appropriately, and so on aren't punishments. You may have spent years already thinking they are, and you actually need to completely reverse that way of thinking.

Find the appropriate carrot-stick ratio that works best for you. Just be careful: Too much of the stick can actually decrease motivation and performance. Make sure you balance anti-rewards with rewards and give yourself a well-deserved pat on the back from time to time as well. Even with the stick method, don't deprive or truly punish yourself. If you don't reach your goal, you can — and should — try again. Stay away from the negative self-talk and make your action plan even sturdier for the next go-round.

Look into an Alternate Future

When you need a motivational boost, close your eyes and imagine what your life will look like in the future — three, six, or 12 months or longer from now — if you were to quit today.

When thinking of this alternate future, ask yourself some questions, such as:

- If you quit now, how will you look in a few months' time? How will you feel?
- What will your health be like? Your cholesterol? Your blood pressure?
- If you went back to your unhealthy lifestyle, how much weight would you gain in the next few months?
- How will your children, significant other, family, and friends be impacted by your decision to quit being healthy?
- Will you feel ashamed of yourself if you quit now?

Make sure you're honest with yourself. Think about how you felt and looked before you began your healthy lifestyle journey and the positive changes you've made so far, and then create questions and scenarios around those things. For example, if you quit now, would you go back to sleeping poorly? Would you feel sick of wearing ill-fitting clothes? Would you feel fatigued?

This motivational tactic forces you to take stock of the life you lived prior to deciding to get healthy and how much worse you would feel if you continued along that unhealthy path. That future can be a very scary place, but the beautiful thing about your future is that it hasn't been decided yet. *You* are in control. So use this glimpse of the future to reinforce your resolve to the point that you feel motivated enough to know that you *will* continue along your healthful journey, and that scary unhealthy future isn't going to be yours.

Visualize Your Healthy Future

You can use visualization to imagine and picture what your healthy future will look like, if you continue to adhere to your current healthy lifestyle overhaul. With *visualization,* you recreate all the images, feelings, and even sounds of a particular event; however, you allow only for a positive outcome, doing away with any negative feelings or thoughts that would normally inhibit your success. This technique works by strengthening the mental pathways used during whatever activity you're visualizing, thus increasing your chances of success.

Top athletes frequently use visualization in the moments, days, and months leading up to a sporting event. Research has shown that those athletes who do visualize perform better in their respective sport than those athletes who don't, meaning that the athletes who practice visualization on a regular basis not only hone their physical skills but also strengthen their mental game.

To visualize, spend five to ten minutes a day (you can split up that time in small bits) and picture the future and what it looks like after you've reached all your goals. To visualize, follow these easy steps:

1. **Close your eyes and take several deep breaths.**

2. **Pick a very positive mental image of a specific future event.**

   The moment doesn't have to be monumental. It can be as simple as spending a day at the beach or achieving a personal athletic goal, but the point is to start with a moment in time that is very specific. For example, you have a beach trip planned with friends, and it'll be the first time that you'll be out in public, in a bathing suit, since committing to a fasting program.

3. **After you're relaxed, imagine the scene playing out with the first step you take.**

   Imagine the confidence you'll feel when you step on the sand for the first time, knowing that you've been fasting, exercising, and living more healthfully for the past three months.

4. **Visualize yourself succeeding.**

   Picture your friends as they ask you what you've been doing that makes you look so lean and sure of yourself. Imagine how you answer their questions. Picture yourself walking along the surf and not feeling like you want to hide your body beneath a swim cover-up or shirt.

Visualization practice isn't the time to focus on any negative thoughts. If you find that a negative thought is creeping in, say to yourself "erase," and then replay the image with a positive outcome. It may take more than one time of saying "erase" for you to finally nix the negative images that pop into your mind, but keep at it. You'll find that over time your visualization will be increasingly positive.

The success rates of people who use visualization show just how powerful the mind really is. If you direct your mind to positive visualization, you can create your ideal future — the future in which you're healthy, confident, and secure. After you picture your ideal future in your mind, you can find that, regardless of your past, attaining that future seems much more doable and not some far-fetched idea that you will never be able to achieve.

Focus on the Positive Feelings

Confident, balanced, energetic, *alive*. Have you experienced any of these positive feelings since you first tried fasting? If you're looking for motivation, focus on a time when you began your journey toward health and remember when you felt good, really good, about your new lifestyle. Maybe it was after successfully completing a fast or turning down dessert or upon receiving a compliment about your glowing skin or waking up truly rested for the first time in years. You felt great, knowing that you successfully completed a day-long fast.

Oftentimes when you lack motivation, you simply are stuck in the moment; the unhealthy lifestyle of your past has a stronger pull and you can't remember when you felt good about making the switch to a healthy lifestyle. Perhaps you don't remember feeling that unhealthy before, and sticking to your current regimen seems much more difficult than not. However, remembering these positive feelings and reliving them can provide a much-needed motivational boost. Because, the truth is, you *have* felt some positive emotions since you began your fasting journey. You just need to spend some time remembering them.

Your memory can play tricks on you. You may think that your once-unhealthy lifestyle wasn't really that bad compared to enduring your current healthy lifestyle. To get your mind back on track and to get motivated, spend some time remembering and reliving the positive feelings that you experienced since you began fasting, anything from remembering when your skinny jeans finally fit to being able to play with your kids without getting tired out.

Take Stock of the Positive Changes You've Experienced

Because you're in the thick of making progress, you may not be able to see the progress you've already made. If so, spend some time taking stock of the positive changes you've experienced since you committed to a fasting method, rather than looking at the progress you *haven't* made (yet).

Notice how much better your clothes fit. Think about how well you've been sleeping lately. Maybe you weren't able to complete a 12-hour fast at the beginning, but now you've worked your way up to a 24-hour fast once a week. If you've been committed to fasting (no matter what method you've chosen), you probably have made progress. You just need to take a moment and figure out what that progress looks like to you, and remember that your progress may not be a plummeting number on the bathroom scale.

If you continue to feel like your motivation is suffering because you aren't seeing the results you want, you may need to reevaluate your goals. If your goals aren't specific enough and aren't measurable from the start (for example, "I'll start fasting and lose weight"), seeing progress can be incredibly difficult. Try revamping your goals to make them more specific and measurable (for example, "I'll lose two pounds a week for the next month by committing to the micro-fasting method, by going for daily walks, and by exercising three times a week"). You'll feel so much more confident in yourself by creating such an assertive, positive goal that it will become much easier to see the progress you're making and keep your end goal in sight.

Be Compassionate with Yourself

Sometimes you just aren't going to feel motivated and you aren't going to have as successful a day or week as you would have liked. Employing negative self-talk and getting down on yourself because you didn't meet your own expectations won't help you in the long-run. When you encounter the rough times, the best thing you can do is be compassionate with yourself.

If you find that you just can't get yourself to complete a fast or that you can't ignore the siren's call of that slice of leftover birthday cake, no matter what, don't be hard on yourself. Think about how you can set yourself up for success and how you *will* set yourself up for success in the future. The next time you're tempted, you can toss the leftover cake in the trash before you have a chance to be tempted by it. Maybe you can plan your post-fast meals better. Or perhaps you can visualize your healthy fit future self, enjoying yourself at the beach. (Refer to the earlier section, "Visualize Your Healthy Future" for how to visualize.)

You're only human. If you don't meet your own expectations, take stock of the situation and figure out what you can do better next time to ensure success. In doing so, you can cultivate compassion for your faults as well as conviction in your inner strength. The next time you're faced with a choice of whether or not to stay on the healthy path, you'll be more likely to stick with it and find the motivation you need.

Get in the Habit of Motivating Yourself

Motivation is a habit, and like all habits, if you want it to become second nature, you must practice it. And practice it on a regular basis.

Set aside 15 to 20 minutes a day to think about your goals, your progress, where you see yourself now, and where you want to be. Find positive affirmations that are meaningful to you and recite them — in your mind, in the car, or in front of a mirror. Some of our favorite affirmations to recite include the following:

- ✔ Every day I am getting healthier and feeling better.
- ✔ I avoid junk food and continue to give my body the nutritious food it craves.
- ✔ Good health is my birthright. Every day I am working to regain that right.
- ✔ I am full of patience, compassion, and strength.
- ✔ My strongest asset is my health, and my daily actions and thoughts invest in that asset.
- ✔ I am so grateful for my health, my family, my friends, and my life.

You don't have to practice motivation in one 20-minute chunk. Practicing motivation may be more effective if you break it up over the course of the day. Try for three or four five-minute sessions throughout the day. You can try any combination of the tactics we discuss in this chapter or others that you've found that work for you. Experiment and find what works best for you! Pretty soon you'll find that motivation is something that comes naturally and effortlessly.

Chapter 16

Ten Ways to Feel Energized When You're Fasting

In This Chapter

▶ Tapping into energy when you're dragging

▶ Drinking water and caffeine

*I*f you're new to fasting, you may feel that eating is one of the best ways to give yourself an energy boost. However, eating often makes people feel a lack of energy because your body releases an influx of insulin after you eat, which aids in digestion by helping your body utilize the glucose and amino acids that it received from the food you ate. No wonder you feel in need of a boost of energy. Your body thinks it's time to nap. However, if you're fasting but still have trouble keeping your energy level high, try employing any combination of these methods. Mix and match, play around, and see which ones work best.

Stand Up and Start Moving

When you lack energy while fasting, you can often blame it not on the absence of food, but on the absence of movement. In general, people are quite sedentary, sitting in front a computer screen, behind a steering wheel, or on the couch. To start feeling energized, take a walk, do a mini workout, stretch.

Even if you work out regularly, regular movement during the day is important. Especially if you sit for long periods of time, make sure you stand up and move. You can do a couple sets of squats, push-ups, or lunges, or you can just walk; it doesn't have to be complicated. Set an alarm to remind yourself to do so for five minutes every hour. Although the activity is short in duration, the movement can improve blood flow and sustain energy levels.

Become a Social Butterfly

If your energy is waning, walk to the nearest office water cooler and chat. Socializing can take your mind off the tiring effect that mental and physical stress has on the body. It's a form of mental exercise that is minimally stressful, boosts brainpower, and staves off fatigue (as long as you aren't socializing with a person who causes you stress in the first place).

Furthermore, being social is good for your overall health. A 2008 study found that talking to another person for just 10 minutes a day improves cognitive functions such as memory, and researchers who conducted a 1999 Harvard study found that people who kept just five social relationships significantly decreased their chances for cognitive performance decline.

Drink Plenty of Water

Water can help you keep your energy level high. For one, dehydration is a sneaky cause of fatigue, and no matter if you're experiencing even a mild case of dehydration, it affects levels of concentration and cognition. If you aren't adequately keeping your body's water level high enough and you enter even a mild state of dehydration, then your body struggles to perform its usual functions, such as sweating, transporting nutrients, and keeping you feeling good.

Spend a week increasing the amount of water you drink (and getting rid of less optimal beverages, such as soda, diet or otherwise, and other sugar-laden drinks), until you reach the recommended amount. We also suggest that during fasting, you actually drink even more fluids than the suggested eight glasses to help transport nutrients throughout your body and get rid of toxins as they're released during the fasting process.

Use Caffeine Wisely

Caffeine can provide just the boost you need to get your day started (or going). Studies have shown that consuming caffeine has a positive effect on physical exertion and mental activity. Whether you're hitting the gym to get in the day's workout or trying to concentrate on a demanding project at work, drinking a cup of coffee or two can help with your performance.

Drinking too much caffeine can be counterproductive, especially if it interferes with your nightly sleeping routine. Keep caffeine consumption to earlier in the day and don't drink more than two cups of coffee (or other healthy caffeinated beverage, such as green or black tea) per day. Also stay away from energy drinks. They're laden with sugar and send your body into a state of hyperactivity, impeding your mental and physical performance.

Breathe In Some Aromatherapy

Smell is the strongest of senses. By utilizing this sense, you can positively affect productivity, brain activity, and energy levels. Here is a list of scents that can give you a positive energy boost when you need it most:

- ✔ Lavender has a calming effect on the mind and improves mood.
- ✔ Citrus (such as lemon or orange) promotes concentration levels.
- ✔ Rosemary increases alertness and memory retention.
- ✔ Peppermint stimulates clear thinking.

Breathing in a few inhalations of these scents, whether you're sniffing some from a few drops on a cotton ball or adding a small amount to a diffuser or mister, can activate your hypothalamus and invigorate your entire body and mind. Try it first thing in the morning or whenever you need a burst of energy anytime throughout the day.

Play a Game

Playing a game can minimize stress and provide a boost of energy. While you're playing a game, your mind doesn't shut down. It stays active but at pleasant and nonstressful levels, which results in stimulating the brain without either overloading it, like when you're doing challenging mental work, or turning it off, such as when you're watching television.

To make the most effective use of this method, set a time limit on the game you decide to play. For instance, you may only play three rounds or ten minutes before returning to whatever you were doing prior to your break. You'll find that your energy levels have been given a healthy boost and you're ready to keep on tackling the day.

Listen to Some of Your Favorite Music

If you're feeling a lag in energy on a fast day, slip on a pair of headphones and listen to music. Try out different kinds of music, too. You may find that while classical music gives you an energy boost, listening to pop music may be a little too distracting for whatever work you're trying to do.

A 2001 study confirmed that listening to music increases the blood flow to the brain's pleasure centers in the same manner that eating food might stimulate pleasure in the brain. An added bonus: Studies have shown that people engaging in creative work reported a heightened sense of creativity while listening to music, making their jobs easier.

Have More Sex More Often

Humans are programmed to enjoy sex and to reap some wonderful health benefits from this intimate act, including an increase in endorphin production. Endorphins, which are a brain chemical, create a sense of well-being and can provide a much-needed boost of energy. Although you may not be able to (or maybe not want to) have sex when you're tired, try to have sex more frequently. By increasing the amount of sex that you do have, you can keep energy levels higher in the long run and keep your partner happier.

Laugh More and Smile

The average child laughs more than 300 times a day. The average adult? Only five times. The act of laughing can make your general outlook on life better. This improvement in perspective stimulates energy, so take the time to identify what gets you giggling. After you know what works best, give laughter a try whenever you need a burst of energy. Furthermore, studies have shown that laughter improves mood, boosts endorphins, and improves immunity.

Get a Better Night's Sleep

Sleeping better the night before to improve your energy levels may seem obvious, but many people sabotage their chances of getting a good night's sleep. In order to sleep soundly — and stave off fatigue the next day — check out the following tips for getting in a quality sleep session:

✔ Establish a sleep routine (for example, take a shower, turn off the TV, drink a cup of tea, read a relaxing book with dimmed lights, and so on).

✔ Don't drink caffeine too late in the evening.

✔ Don't drink alcohol too close to bedtime and don't use it to fall asleep.

✔ Turn off electronics and other gadgets, such as cellphones or tablets, an hour or two before bed.

✔ Use blackout curtains to keep the room dark throughout the night.

✔ Keep your bedroom cool — not too warm but not frigid.

Index

About the Authors

Kellyann Petrucci, MD, earned her BA from Temple University, hosted her alma mater's Department of Public Health Intern Program, and mentored students entering the health field. She earned her MS degree from St. Joseph's University and Doctor of Chiropractic degree from Logan College of Chiropractic — University Programs, where she served as the Postgraduate Chairperson. Enrolled in postgraduate coursework in Europe, she also studied naturopathic medicine at the College of Naturopathic Medicine, London. She is one of the few practitioners in the United States certified in biological medicine by the esteemed Dr. Thomas Rau, of the Paracelsus Klinik Lustmuhle, Switzerland.

During her many years as a doctor/consultant at her thriving nutrition-based practice in the Philadelphia area, she helped dozens of patients overcome major health issues while building the strongest, healthiest body possible. With years of research and observation, Kellyann learned that feeling — and looking — good came down to simple principles and food values that made an astonishing difference in people's lives. "Overall health is about reprogramming the body to get back to the basics — to learn how to eat the way human bodies were designed to eat," she says. She found the principles of living Paleo to be the key for those who wished to open the door to losing weight, boosting immunity, and fighting aging. With the hundreds of Paleo successes she's seen thus far, Kellyann is committed more than ever to continuing to spread the Paleo lifestyle message.

She has written several health and lifestyle books including *Living Paleo For Dummies, Paleo Cookbook For Dummies, Paleo Workouts For Dummies, and Boost Your Immunity For Dummies* (all with John Wiley & Sons, Inc.). She appears on various news streams nationally and conducts workshops and seminars worldwide to help people feel — and look   their best. She also is the author of the website www.drkellyann.com and gives daily news, tips, and inspiration on twitter@drkellyann.

With her national Paleo door-to-door home delivery food service, www.livingpaleofoods.com, the busy mother of two young sons is committed to making a Paleo lifestyle convenient for everyone, including the extremely busy.

Pat Flynn is a fitness minimalist who wants to help people eat and exercise more deliberately. He believes the secret to a good exercise is simplicity, and that any dietary or fitness regimen will improve in direct ratio to the number of things kept out of it that shouldn't be there.

Pat is the founder of www.chroniclesofstrength.com, a health and wellness blog focused on helping people find clarity in the world of weights through a "less is more" approach to fitness. Pat strips diet and exercise down to its fewest and most fundamental components, helping you to separate the gold from the garbage and get going with what actually works for forging a leaner, harder, and healthier physique.

Pat writes mostly on kettlebell training for strength, mobility, and fat loss. He also talks a lot on intermittent fasting, hormone optimization, sex, health, longevity, supplementation, and any other topic that he believes his readers will find somewhat useful. For a free guide on kettlebell training for strength and fat loss, visit his website. He also offers private online coaching.

Dedication

Kellyann: I dedicate this book to my parents John and El Petrucci. They set such a high standard for healthy living in my home growing up, which I'm so grateful.

Now in their late seventies, they're a pure example of the payoff when you chose to live your life physically active, flood your mind with optimism, and are mindful of healthy nutrition. They're as active as anyone in their forties, and everyday still continues to be an adventure. My mother, a beautiful artist, spends her days painting and taking art classes. My father thinks nothing of walking 18 holes on the golf course, carrying his bag — with the biggest smile on his face the entire time. A few times a week they *bust it up* in my sister's health center, doing metabolic/strength training in the absolute awe of everyone around them. They *truly* are enjoying their life.

This attitude does transcend. I think my sister and I (she's a doc as well) have had something to do with their healthy lifestyle, and we certainly have made an impact. But really, it's the other way around. My parents' lifestyle practices etched an indelible scar that has transcended through their kids. My sister and I became doctors, practicing wellness principles. My younger brother has a black belt in tae kwon do and has been a jujitsu instructor for more than 20 years. My older brother is a competitive cyclist in all disciplines and competes throughout the country. He's even a former three-time state champion. We all have taken on healthy lifestyle practices because of our parents' examples. Being a good role model can make a difference for future generations. I'm forever grateful I was fortunate enough to have that — thanks to John and El.

Pat: I dedicate this book to Christine Mooney. I love you. And to Roan. I love you too.

Authors' Acknowledgments

Kellyann: I was super lucky to have Pat Flynn as my co-author on this project. We first met at a mastermind group and became instant friends. We found that our values and vision for health and wellness were exceedingly congruent, and we knew this book had to be. I call Pat the "Mark Twain of Fitness" because of his great intellect, wit, and charm. These attributes are rounded by the fact he harbors a unique philosophy on how to exercise and live more deliberately, which makes him the fitness guru to so many. I'm appreciative to have collaborated with him and to have become such great friends.

If anyone has ever given you a shot in life, you'll know why I have such deep gratitude for my agent Bill Gladstone of Waterside Productions. He gave me my first big break purely from instinct, and I am forever thankful for his faith and intuition. To Margot Hutchinson of Waterside Productions who was on my side, pitching from the beginning, who is now more than an agent, but has become special in my life.

To my colleagues at Wiley, Acquisition Editor Tracy Boggier who has always been incredibly responsive and always in my court and my Project Editor and Copy Editor Chad Sievers, thanks for lending your talents to build this book. Thanks also to Laura Bollinger for her technical review.

Pat: The lovely and brilliant Dr. Petrucci deserves my first acknowledgement and by a significant margin. This book wouldn't have been if it weren't for her, and I couldn't have asked for a more capable partner. Her brain is huge and I would not be surprised if it weighed near to four pounds. Her passion to help others in their quest for health, strength, and longevity is very close to psychotic. And her ability to actually do so is bewildering, if not downright magical, and it wouldn't surprise me to hear that she has some magic elf in her. Nonetheless, she is wonderful woman, charming as a waterfall, and overflowing with radiance. I suspect that she knows more about healthy living than the person who invented it, and I would without hesitation entrust to her care my very own sweet and tender grandmother and not worry once about phoning for the hearse.

My second acknowledgement goes to that very same sweet and tender grandmother. My third to my mother, fourth to my father, and fifth to my grandfather. These are in no order of importance, mind you, merely just granting them admission as they applied. My sixth acknowledgement goes to Chad Sievers, my project editor and copy editor. I give my seventh acknowledgement to my two dogs, Lola and Chewie, who are of the St. Bernard breed and drool quite a bit and for teaching me everything I know about quantum mechanics. [And then I said, "That's no St. Bernard, that's my mom!"]. My next acknowledgement goes to the whole of The Dragon Gym — Somnath Sikdar, Lonnie Beck, Diana Volante, Chris Taylor, and a few other people here and there whose names and faces escape me at the moment.

My next acknowledgement goes to my agent, Margot. Thank you for selling me. I realize that must have been absurdly difficult.

I am giving my second to last acknowledgement to all of my readers and followers at www.chroniclesofstrength.com. I couldn't do what I do and lead such a posh and extravagant lifestyle if it weren't for all of you giving me your money. So thanks for that.

My last acknowledgement goes out to all the rest of my friends in this world. You know who you are, and I will be sending both of you a signed copy of this book.

Publisher's Acknowledgments

Acquisitions Editor: Tracy Boggier

Project Editor: Chad R. Sievers

Copy Editor: Chad R. Sievers

Technical Editor: Laura Bollinger

Art Coordinator: Alicia B. South

Project Coordinator: Sheree Montgomery

Photographer: Rebekah Ulmer

Illustrator: Elizabeth Kurtzman

Cover Photos: © Brian Jackson/Alamy